Barb's Miracle

How Barb Tarbox
Transformed Her Deadly
Cancer into a
Lifesaving Crusade

Images by Greg Southam
Words by David Staples

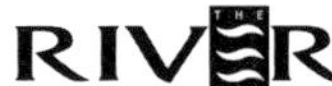
RIVER

River Books and The Books Collective acknowledge the ongoing support of the Canada Council for the Arts and the Alberta Foundation for the Arts and the Edmonton Arts Council for our publishing programme.

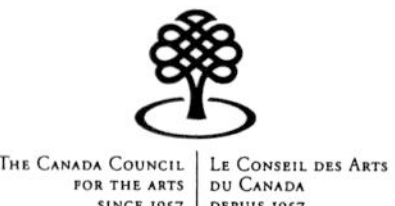

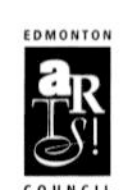

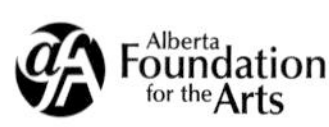

Support and promotional assistance for this book, and for Barb Tarbox's campaign in general, have been provided by the Alberta Alcoholism and Drug Abuse Commission (AADAC), the Alberta Lung Association, ASH, and Mile Zero Consulting. It is not possible to thank individually all those who supported Barb Tarbox's campaign, Barb herself, or the publication of this book, but we extend to each of you (you know who you are) our thanks and gratitude.

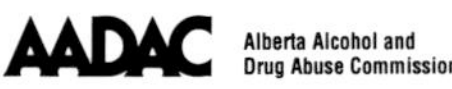

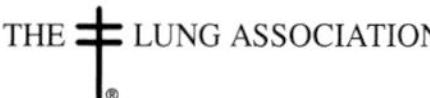

Editors for the press: Candas Jane Dorsey & Timothy J. Anderson.
Cover and inside design by John Luckhurst / GDL, Edmonton.
All photos by Greg Southam except photos on page 7 courtesy Pat Tarbox.
The text was set by John Luckhurst of GDL in *Minion*, a typeface adapted from traditional font designs dating from as early as the 1500s, and copyrighted in 1989 and 1991 by Adobe type designer Robert Slimbach. The Books Collective is working to phase out our use of paper produced from ancient forests (for more information on Ancient Forest Friendly publishing, see Markets Initiative at www.oldgrowthfree.com). To this end, this book was printed and bound in Canada on Jenson Satin 80lb text, a stock with 10% post-consumer recycled content, with vegetable based inks, by Friesen's Printing.

National Library of Canada Cataloguing in Publication

Southam, Greg, 1959-
Barb's miracle : how Barb Tarbox transformed her deadly cancer into a lifesaving crusade / images by Greg Southam ; words by David Staples.

ISBN 1-894880-02-1 (bound).—ISBN 1-894880-03-X (pbk.)

1. Tarbox, Barb, 1961-2003. 2. Antismoking movement—Canada. 3. Cancer—Patients—Canada—Biography. I. Staples, David, 1962- II. Title.

RC265.6.T37S68 2004 363.4'092 C2004-902384-5

Dedications

From David Staples. For Lily, who is my miracle.

From Greg Southam. My loving wife Jennifer and my parents Doug and Isabelle, for their constant support.

Acknowledgments

We both owe a huge debt to Tracy Mueller and Pat Tarbox for their dedication to Barb's vision and for their friendship. Donna Gingera put in as much work as anyone on behalf of Barb. We'd also like to thank our editors at the *Edmonton Journal*, Linda Hughes, Allan Mayer, Roy Wood, Ian Scott, Neil Smalian, Giles Gherson, Bob Bell and Brian Tucker, who supported and guided us throughout the project. Thanks also to Lloyd Carr at AADAC, Les Hagen at ASH, Randy Mark, Terry Elniski, Bob Todrick of McBain Camera, Craig Marler, Gord Deeks, Dr. Ross Halperin, Dr. Douglas Fonteyne, Dr. Martin Palmer, Marilyn Schmidt, John Luckhurst at GDL, Susan Shaw, and all the others who kindly gave time and expertise to this project. Finally, thanks to Candas Jane Dorsey and Timothy J. Anderson of River Books, whose belief in this project was indispensible.

Published in Canada by River Books, an imprint of The Books Collective

214-21, 10405 Jasper Avenue
Edmonton, Alberta T5J 3S2

Telephone (780) 448-0590
Fax (780) 448-0640
E-mail: admin@bookscollective.com
Website: www.bookscollective.com

Introduction

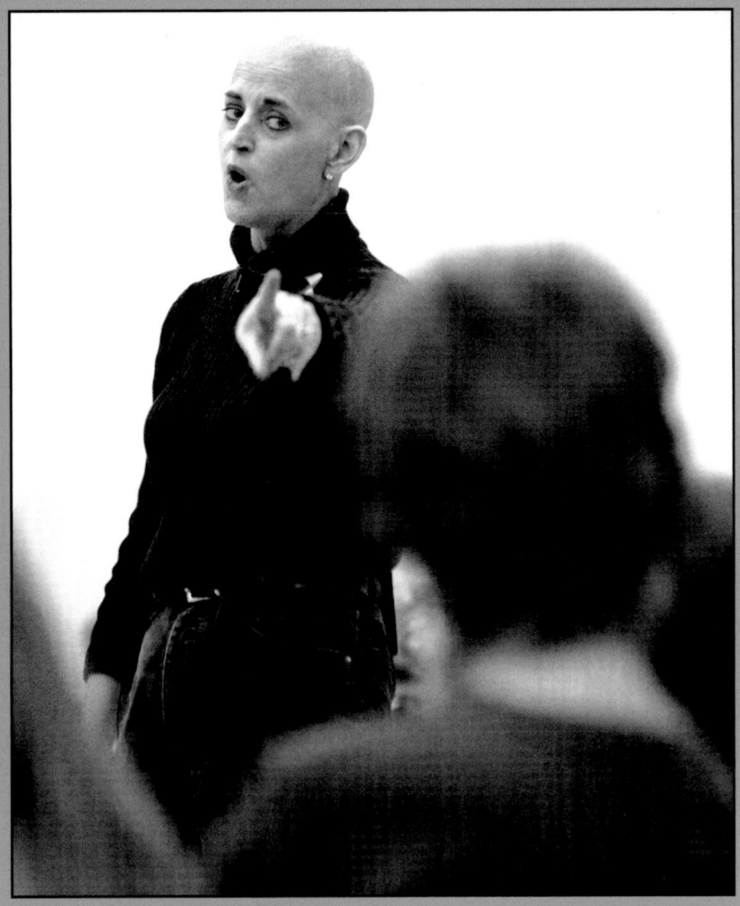

Blessed are those who hunger and thirst for righteousness, for they will be filled.

Matthew 5:6

In the winter of 2003, Barb Tarbox went on a journey that led to her healing and ended in her death. I was Barb's unlikely companion on her final passage. For me, for my colleague, photographer Greg Southam, for everyone who traveled with Barb, it was a time of tears and controversy, darkness and discovery, and one peculiar miracle.

You may well have heard about the public part of Barb's story. Over a six-month period, from November 2002 to April 2003, she staged the most aggressive, unrelenting and effective anti-smoking campaign that North America has ever seen. She spoke to more than 50,000 students at schools across Canada about her 30-year smoking habit and the cancerous tumours it had ignited in her lungs and brain.

"Look at me!" she cried out at school after school. "Remember this face and that smoking killed me!"

Barb got her wish. She went from being an unknown housewife in out-of-the-way Edmonton, Alberta, to a crusader of international renown. She became the spokesperson for the Alberta government's anti-smoking campaign, one with unparalleled success. In a survey, 94 per cent of respondents recalled Barb's TV ads; by comparison, the second most successful anti-smoking ad campaign, a famous series of TV announcements featuring a Californian woman who had to smoke through the breathing hole in her neck, had an 80 per cent audience recall. From March 2002 to March 2003, cigarette sales in Alberta dropped 24.4 per cent, partly due to a tax increase, but also due to Barb.

At the height of her crusade, politicians at Edmonton's City Hall, the Alberta Legislature and the House of Commons in Ottawa gave Barb standing ovations. She shook hands with then prime minister Jean Chrétien. Governor General Adrienne Clarkson gave the Meritorious Service Award to her posthumously. The Montel Williams show in New York broadcast an hour-long special on her.

"I am sure once people see Barb, they will be moved to change their lives," said Williams, himself an ex-smoker. "The day we taped the show in our studio, members of our audience walked out, leaving behind full packs of cigarettes on their chairs."

I wept a dozen times for Barb during her crusade. I wept again writing this book. But, as I said earlier, I was an unlikely companion for her.

I'm a newspaper journalist, and I work to be objective and skeptical, qualities essential to succeeding at my craft. Reporters are forever talking to people who want to use us to get out their message. The charming ones seduce us with their wit and persuasion. The angry ones bash away, calling us idiots if we don't agree with every one of their points. But it's not our job to agree, it's our job to be even-handed and fair, and the surest way to do that is to maintain distance from our subjects.

Barb noticed my aloof manner from the start, remarking to her best friend Tracy Mueller that she didn't know what to make of me, that I wasn't like everyone else — the kids, the teachers, and many of the TV and radio reporters — who'd immediately embraced her and told her how wonderful she was.

Throughout my time with Barb, I probed her motives and challenged her point of view. She enjoyed the media celebrity her crusade brought her, but my unending questions disturbed her, so much so that at one point she threatened to end our relationship, cutting out not just me, but also Greg.

I was an unlikely companion for Barb in one other way, as well, at least if you're inclined to believe what Father Mike Mireau said at Barb's funeral in May 2003. He told the mourners that there is a God, that Jesus was his son, and that at the end of Barb's life, God chose to work a miracle through her, creating in Barb an image of Jesus, his mission, his suffering and his love.

"I'm willing to stand here and stake my reputation as a priest on my conviction that what we have witnessed with Barb is a miracle," Father Mike said. "It's God showing up in our lives, bringing triumph out of tragedy, bringing life out of death."

While Barb herself was a true believer, I'm agnostic, which means I've yet to be convinced whether or not God exists. I could well be put into that camp of thinkers that the noted Christian apologist C.S. Lewis referred to as *modern materialists*, not given to accepting God, hell, heaven or miracles.

"Whatever experiences we may have, we shall not regard them as miraculous if we already hold a philosophy which excludes the supernatural," Lewis wrote. "Any event which is claimed as a miracle is, in the last resort, an experience received from the senses; and the senses are not infallible. We can always say we have been the victims of an illusion. . . If we disbelieve in the supernatural that is what we always shall say."

For example, Lewis said, if the world ended in the Apocalypse described in the Bible, if heaven rolled up, the great white throne appeared, and a person such as me found himself hurled into the Lake of Fire, I would tell myself it was all a hallucination, even as I burned forevermore.

So it could well be that a miracle occurred with Barb, just as Father Mike said it did, and I was so fixated on framing everything within my rationalist, journalistic worldview that I missed it.

Except that's not what happened.

In the final months of Barb's life, I did witness something.

I won't say what that miracle was, not here. My understanding of it unfolded over the months of her messy, inspiring, flawed and madcap crusade; it needs to be explained in that context. But I feel compelled to write this book, to share the good news, so to speak, that a light shone from the darkness of an agonizing cancer death.

And though I was an unlikely companion for Barb, perhaps I was also the right one. How much the better to have her miracle witnessed by a doubter, someone to probe the fault lines, question everything, and take voluminous notes, filling 26 notebooks, and more than 2,000 scribbled pages?

If a miracle is to be believed, it must withstand scrutiny. This one does.

DAVID STAPLES
Edmonton, Alberta, Canada
May 18, 2004

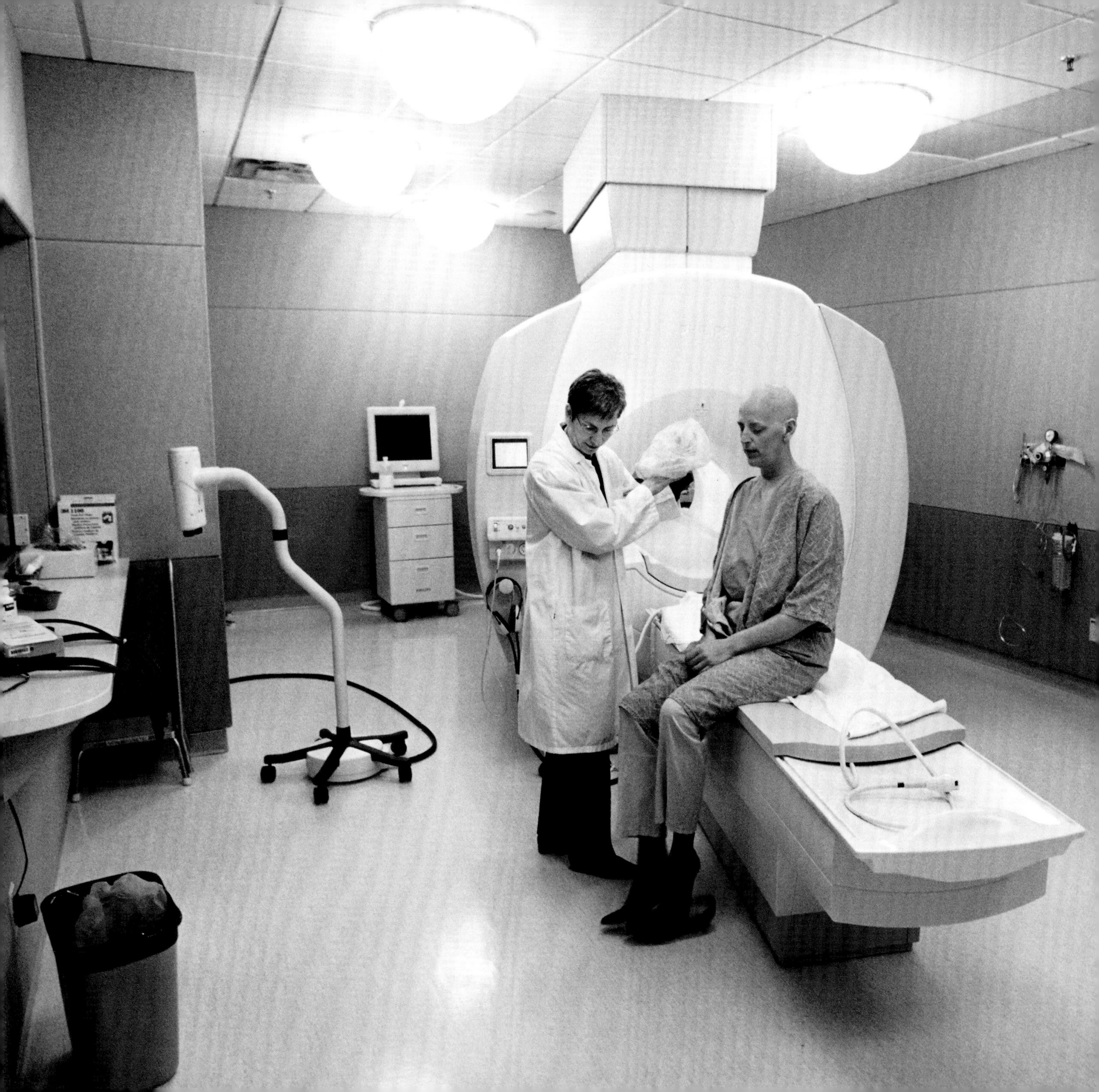

November

2 0 0 2

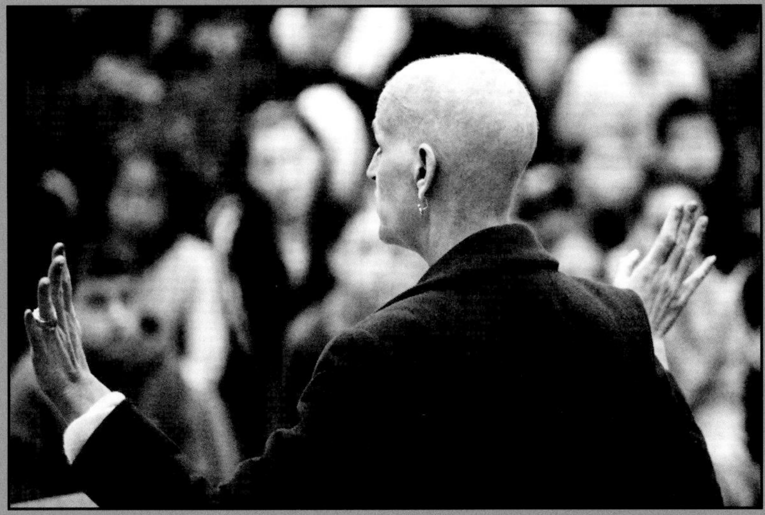

It is only when we truly know and understand that we have a limited time on earth — and that we have no way of knowing when our time is up — that we will be begin to live each day to the fullest, as if it was the only one we had.

Dr. Elisabeth Kübler-Ross

Wednesday, November 27. I met Barb Tarbox at her home, a plain bungalow in a modest city suburb of winding roads, cul-de-sacs and double garages. First impression? A tall, slender woman, sharp, striking features, large blue eyes, thick lashes, layered-on make-up over pale skin, a hat to cover her bald head.

She'd just had her first really bad day, she told me, and it had left her frightened but unbowed. She was determined to keep delivering her anti-smoking message to students, she said. "If I was to lay down right now, I'd probably die. That's what people do."

Her goal was to speak to 7,000 kids by mid-December, right about the time she expected her cancer to lay her low.

Ever since she'd spoken at her first school at the end of October, things had been extremely busy, she said. Schools were constantly calling her or her best friend Tracy Mueller to set up a time for her presentation. "They ask me, 'How much?' I don't charge anything for this. I refuse. *I refuse.* I will never accept anything."

So her crusade wasn't about money, not that I expected it would be. But why then? Why do this strange thing?

Put yourself in her place. You're only 41 years old, but you've been diagnosed with Stage IV cancer, inoperable tumours in your lungs and brain and on your heart. The brain tumour is most likely to kill you. That will probably take just a few months, doctors suspect: by Christmas 2002 or not much later. The tumour on the heart is more unpredictable, though; it could trigger cardiac arrest. Any second could be your last.

Already, you feel death's grip. You have no appetite. Your head throbs. Your bowels are wracked with diarrhea. You ache, as the tumours eat through organs and bone. Your energy has never been lower. It's like the worst flu you've ever had, only it never gets better, only worse. Why not just curl up on the couch in a pitiful ball of sadness? And, once you're done with your grieving — if you ever do get done — why not retreat into the comforting embrace of your closest family and friends? That's what everybody does when they find out they have terminal cancer, is it not?

I'd never heard of anyone doing what Barb was embarking upon, heading out to schools, showing off her radiation-scarred bald head and withered body, crying out to teenagers about the evils of a 30-year addiction to cigarettes.

The uniqueness of Barb's quest made me curious about her motives, so in this first interview with her, I delved into her background, looking for clues.

Barb's family came from northern Ireland. Her parents Harold and Lylia Ditty married there, then immigrated to Canada in 1952, Harold to work as an Edmonton city police officer, Lylia as a nurse. Barb was born April 10, 1961, the second of two children. She grew up to be tall and slender like her dad, gregarious like her mother.

Both parents smoked. Harold quit when he was 40, after he had his first major heart attack. His heart never was strong again. He died from another heart attack at age 67.

When Barb was 11, she stole her first cigarette from her mother's purse. Smoking it made her throw up, but she kept at it. She quickly came to like both the taste of the cigarette and the new friends that smoking brought her. At school, she was one of the pretty, high-status girls, and was known for her love of sports, drama class and socializing. But Barb didn't feel on top of things herself. She smoked du Maurier because they were the popular brand, and that's what it was all about for Barb: popularity.

"Everybody was smoking and there was a lot of peer pressure," Barb told me. "It was all about being cool. I caved right in."

A great wave of young North American women started smoking in the 1970s, partly inspired by the cigarette industry's clever use of women's liberation themes: *You've come a long way, baby!*

For Barb, liberation meant pooling her money with girlfriends to buy cigarettes, then hiding them in the plastic barrel from her *Barrel of Monkeys* game. By grade seven, she smoked every day behind her garage. When her mom caught Barb, she grounded her, but Barb was unrepentant.

"*You* smoke," the 11-year-old girl shot back.

By grade nine, Barb was smoking a pack a day. She lost her wind and her interest in sports. One Christmas, her parents got her skis. Barb didn't have the heart to tell them that she no longer had the lung capacity to make it down the hill.

After graduating from high school in 1979, Barb traveled and did some modeling work in Ireland and England. By then, she was smoking two packs a day. She was the kind of smoker who would light up a new cigarette before she'd finished the old one. She never had a boyfriend who didn't smoke. She stopped going to places where she couldn't smoke. If she had a coffee, she had to smoke; after a meal, she had to smoke.

In the fall of 1982, Barb returned home from Europe to find her mom, 57 years old now, dying of lung cancer. Lylia had smoked for 40 years. The cancer spread to her pancreas, brain, bones and liver. Finally, it put her in a coma.

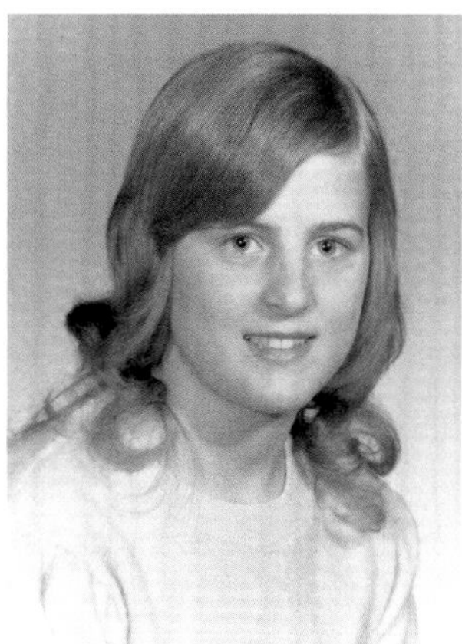

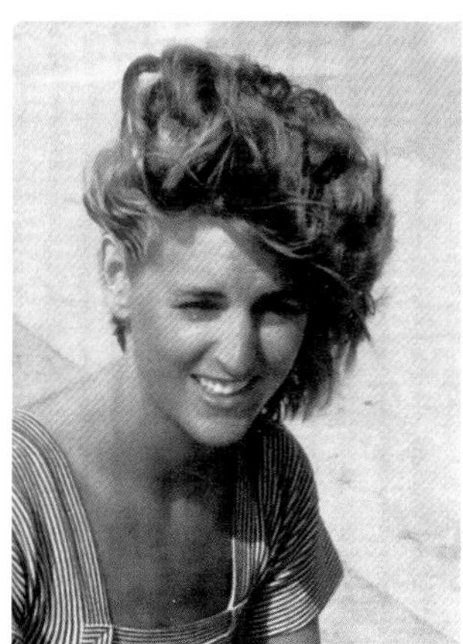

Barb first smoked in grade six (left). By her modeling days (centre) she was smoking two packs a day.

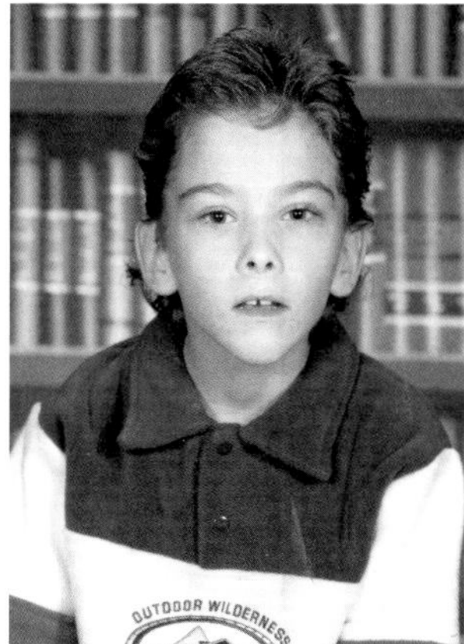

Barb's son Michael, (right) who died at age eight from a congenital heart defect, possibly related to Barb's smoking.

Barb visited her mother daily in the hospital, which is where Lylia's physician, Dr. Tony Fields, noticed that the daughter was a smoker, too.

Fields sat Barb down. "If you don't quit, I'm going to see you here in 20 years," he said.

It was now 19 years later.

She'd been too stressed out to quit when her mom was dying. She had also thought to herself that 20 years was a long time. Surely there'd be a cure for cancer by then.

She had tried quitting, but was always back smoking in a day or two. She went on the nicotine patch, but she cheated and smoked while wearing it.

After Lylia's death, Barb found work in Edmonton as a waitress at restaurants and lounges. She met her future husband, Pat Tarbox, in October, 1983. He was a lounge manager, a tall, dashing and driven young man. Barb followed Pat as he went from job to job in the unstable hospitality industry, moving across Canada and down into the Caribbean. The two married in February 1987.

On December 14, 1990, Barb gave birth to twins, Patrick and Michael. They were born three months prematurely, each weighing two pounds, two ounces. Two weeks later, an infection went around the neonatal ward. It killed tiny Patrick; Michael survived.

Michael was a beautiful child, large round eyes, curly hair, but he proved to be extremely difficult. Screaming fits were the norm. Any little thing set him off — if there was a noise, if someone took him upstairs, if someone took his photograph. As he grew, Barb and Pat noticed he had trouble with co-ordination. He was slow to learn any speech. At last, he was diagnosed as autistic.

Michael's condition brought out strength in Barb that her family and friends had never seen before. His great need tested her, but she found it in herself to cope. She and Pat came to believe that it was fated, that God would not have given them such a test if they couldn't handle it.

Michael woke up every morning at 4:00 a.m., so Barb did too, rising before the sun, going to bed early in the evening. She doted on him. He loved Christmas so much that as soon as Halloween was over, she would put up Christmas decorations.

In an early education program, Barb noticed that Michael wasn't screaming so much. He seemed to be following instructions. The teachers had a habit of singing to the children. Barb wondered if there was a link. She sang to Michael everywhere they went, down the aisles at supermarkets, at home. She even sang to Pat if Michael was around: *Pat, O Pat, get up or you will be late for work, O Pat.*

Over the next 18 months, Michael learned to talk by mimicking her singing. He also started to speak with some emotional nuance, rare for an autistic child. When he reached school age, he went into a special needs program at Malcolm Tweddle school. Barb was there every day as well, with her new and healthy baby, her cherub of a daughter, Mackenzie, born February 17, 1993.

The one thing Barb wouldn't do for Michael was quit smoking. He would rail on about how he hated his mom and dad smoking, repeating this line endlessly. But cigarettes kept Barb going.

In 1998, Michael became increasingly pale and listless. On December 23 that year, he and Mackenzie were dancing in the living room when Michael

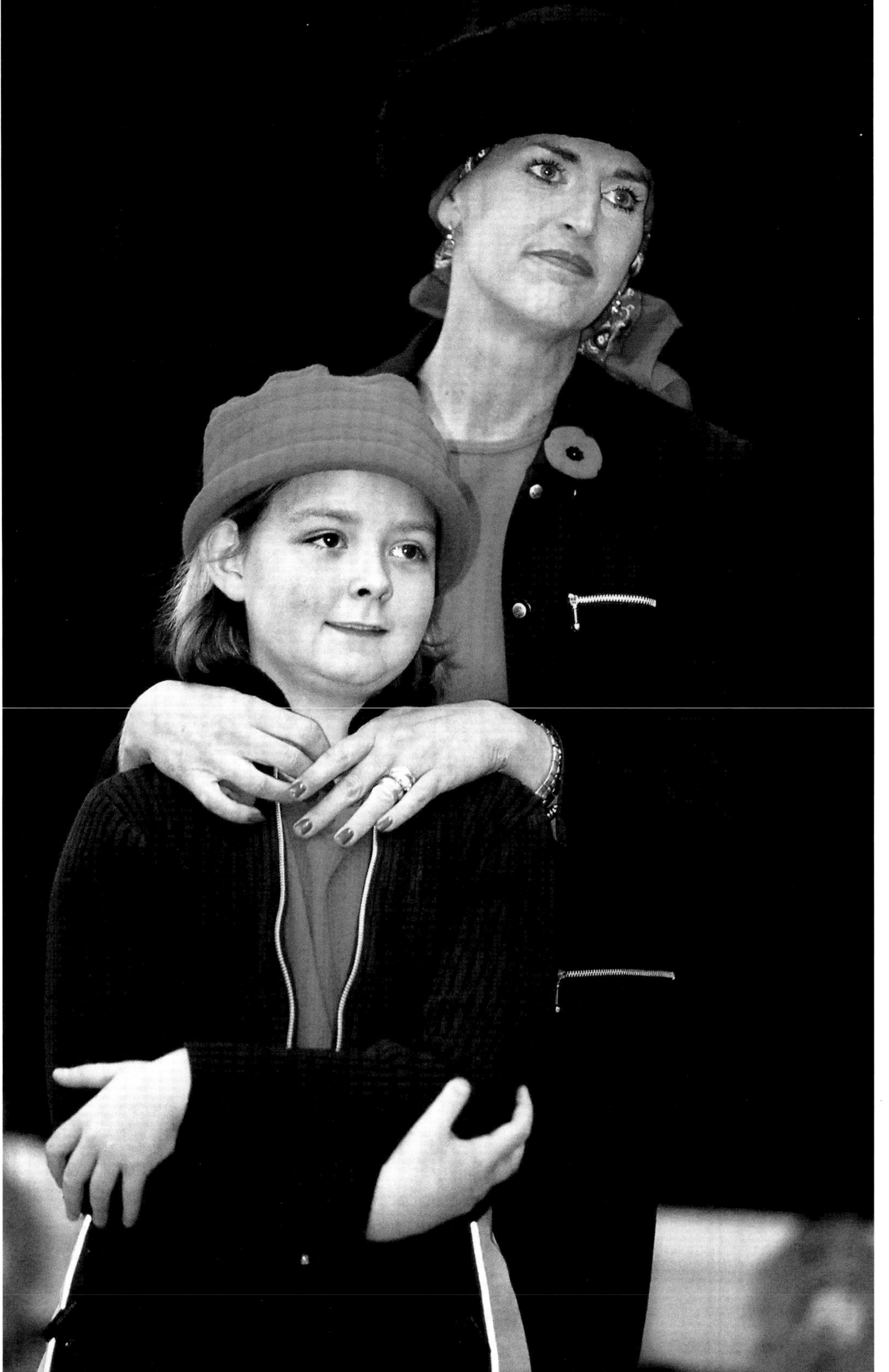

November 11, 2002 - Barb is recognized during an assembly at Malcolm Tweddle school for all the work she put into raising money for the Kids for Cancer run. Mackenzie ran to the front of the auditorium to be with her mother.

suddenly collapsed. Pat called 911 but couldn't get through. He picked up his son, grabbed little Mackenzie and rushed to the hospital. Nothing could be done. Michael died of a heart attack, the victim of a rare and undetected congenital heart defect. He was eight years old.

To cope, Pat got right back to work. Barb also got back at it, focusing more on Mackenzie and volunteering, reading with sick children so they could keep up in their studies. To her friends, it seemed that Barb had started a search for something. She always drove Mackenzie to school, then met with other moms for coffee. She would ask them what they had dreamed the night before, then go home and analyze their dreams, writing out reports, which she would hand back to the other moms at the end of the day. She started trying out different churches.

After Michael's death, Pat fulfilled a promise he'd made to his son and quit smoking. Barb saw smoking was aging her, discolouring her fingers, but still continued her two-pack-a-day habit. She realized her smoking might have consequences, though, so twice a year went in to have her chest X-rayed as a precaution.

Fast forward to August 2002. She was feeling great, with double the energy of most people. She didn't have a cough. Yet an abnormality was found in her X-ray. It looked like a fold in the skin, nothing serious perhaps, but worrisome enough that Barb decided to pay $450 for an immediate private CT scan. The scan revealed three tumours: one in her lung, one on a bronchial tube, one on her heart. They were advanced and inoperable.

Cancer is an uncontrolled abnormal growth of immature cells, which create a mass known as a tumour. Cells can break away from this tumour, enter the bloodstream and spread throughout the body. This is how Barb's cancer had spread from her lungs.

She was sent to Edmonton's main cancer treatment hospital, the Cross Cancer Institute, where she was put under the care of radiologist Dr. Ross Halperin and chemotherapist Dr. Martin Palmer. The doctors hoped the tumours were still relatively small and contained, so that treatment might still save her.

Of the 100 new patients that come to Halperin with inoperable lung cancer every year, 90 die in short order. Of the remaining ten, eight have their cancer return after treatment and die within five years. Only two make it to the five year mark and are considered cured.

At an appointment in early September, Barb complained of smelling a strange scent. Halperin feared the cancer had moved to her brain, bringing on olfactory hallucinations. He confirmed this on September 19 with a scan. Barb had a two-centimetre-long tumour in her lower temporal lobe.

Four days later, Halperin broke the news to her.

In doing this job, Halperin tries to feel sympathy for his patients, but not empathy. He doesn't want to feel what they feel, as it would tear him apart. With Barb, though, it was different. She was so young and had such an engaging personality that Halperin had trouble containing his emotions. Tears glistened in his eyes when he met her.

"Barb," he said, "you're now Stage IV terminal. You've got a massive tumour in your brain. You have very little time left now."

"What if I quit smoking now?" Barb asked at once.

"Will that help?"

No, Halperin said. Quitting might help ease her breathing as her cancer advanced, but it wouldn't give her any extra time, or any more hope.

Barb put her hand on Halperin's shoulder. "I'm Irish!" she said. "I'm never going to stop fighting."

When Barb told Mackenzie the news, the two fell to the floor, holding each other, weeping. "Mommy, how many days am I going to have with you?" the nine-year-old asked.

Barb promised she would make it to Christmas, and made Mackenzie promise that she would never smoke.

Untreated, a person with a brain tumour like the one Barb had lives one or two months on average. With treatment, that stretches to six months.

In early October, Barb had ten sessions of radiation therapy. A plastic mask was made of her face, designed to fit snugly so she could be firmly pinned down as the radiation was directed at the tumour.

After her treatment, Barb's hair started to fall out. Right then, she decided to set an example for Mackenzie, to show how a negative could be turned into a positive. Mother and daughter cut off the remainder of Barb's hair, washed it, and hung it up in their backyard tree. Barb knew that birds love hair for their nests. The next day, when Barb and Mackenzie checked, all the hair was gone.

At school, Mackenzie wrote an essay about her mom: "When I was just a little girl I was always taught to look at things on the bright side. I have grown up having my mom there beside me. Always there when I was sick and always in a good mood. Now she has cancer and it's the other way around and I'm taking care of her at difficult times, but she's always there. When I don't have courage, she gives me courage. When I don't have strength, she gives me strength. At any time in the world she's always here. I think my mom should get a billion of awards for being the best."

Knowing that the cancer would soon take away her appetite, Barb ate double portions of all her favourite foods: Irish stew, shepherd's pie, steak, pork chops, potatoes.

In mid-November, Barb, Pat and friends went out to her favourite Greek restaurant, Grub Med, and ordered her favourite supper — lamb, potatoes and salad. She could eat only a few bites. The food nauseated her. Her lack of hunger worried her friends, which made Barb feel even worse. She always loved a good time, "life and laughter," as she put it. She hated bringing down everyone else.

The first truly bad day was Monday, November 25. Barb had been invited to speak at an out-of-town school, but felt too weak and dizzy to go.

"To hell with this!" she yelled out. "Why is it doing it to me? It's not December. I have a lot of commitments!"

It turned out that Barb was severely dehydrated. At the hospital, she was hooked up to intravenous fluids and soon felt better.

The public part of Barb's final days started in September, when she decided to raise money by participating in the annual Kids for Cancer run at Malcolm Tweddle school. She shared her plan to run with her friend Tracy Mueller, the controller at Team Ford, a large local car dealership. Tracy thought the

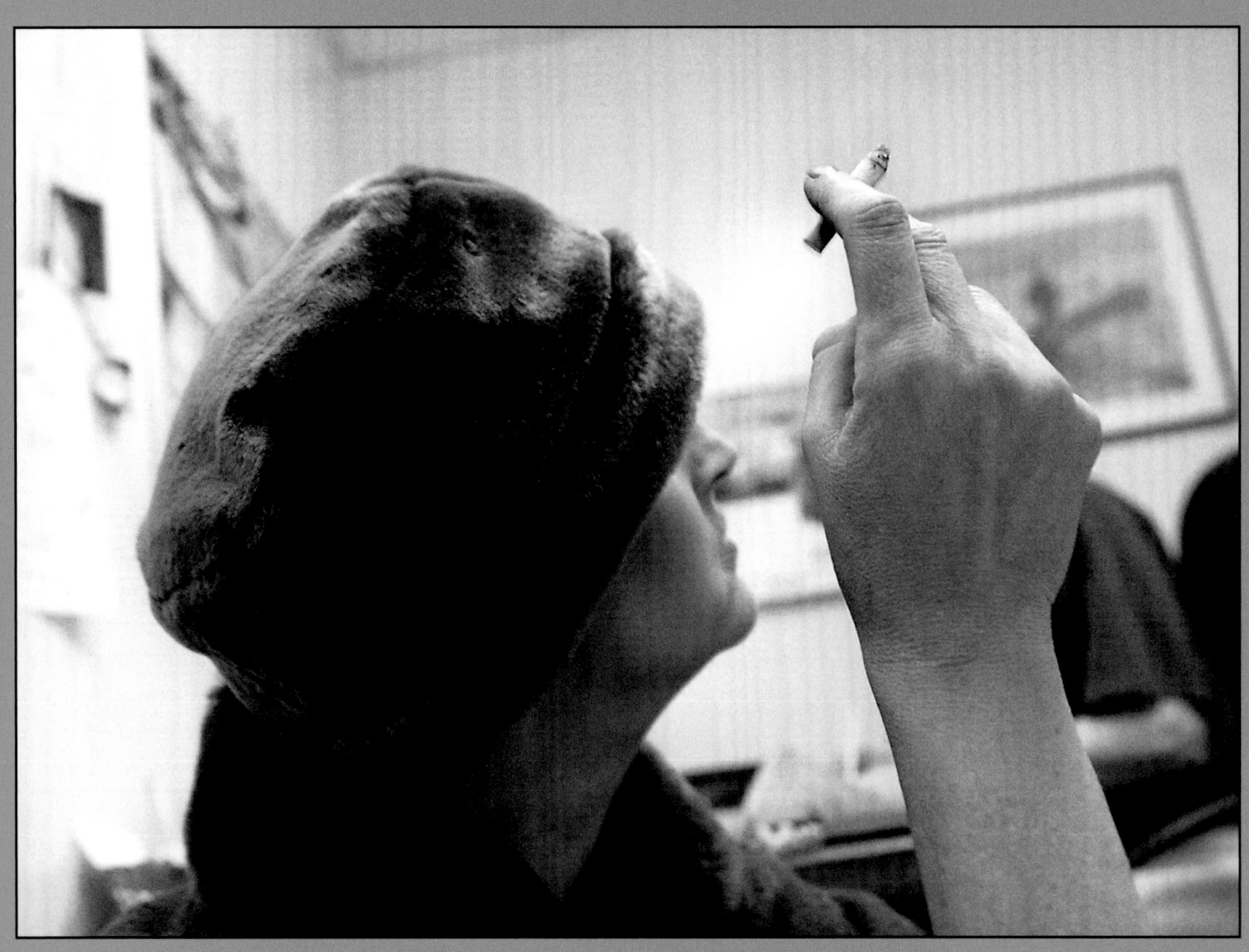

Barb enjoys a cigarette in the back room of her favourite restaurant, Grub Med.

media might be interested in Barb's story, so she called up a few reporters. Sure enough, two TV stations and two newspaper reporters turned out, including Cathy Lord from the *Edmonton Journal.* Barb wowed them with her positive attitude and anti-smoking passion. One cameraman wept. Right then, Tracy had an inkling; she knew it was hard to get the media out for anything, but they had come to see Barb and loved her.

"This is going to be something big," Tracy told Barb.

Barb thought Tracy meant she might get the chance to talk at some big Edmonton schools, maybe even travel to a town outside the city.

In late October, Barb's niece Ashley asked her if she would speak to Ashley's class at T.D. Baker junior high school. Barb agreed, though she was nervous about public speaking. She wrote out her speech and practiced it. On October 29, she read it to a class of 30 kids.

"I'm Barb Tarbox and I'm here today to talk to you about smoking and cancer and overcoming obstacles and adversity that can appear in your life," she started out. "But by using positive energy and thoughts you can overcome all negatives. My greatest obstacle that I have grows within me. I have been a smoker for nearly 30 years. I wish I had listened to my friends when I was in grade seven, as they kept saying, 'Barb, quit smoking!' But now at age 41, which I can assure you is still very young, I am dying of lung cancer. I have very little time left."

Barb hardly strayed from the text, but still grabbed attention by taking off her hat to show off her bald head, by passing around her radiation mask, the ghastly ornament of her therapy, and by having the kids feel her cold hands.

"I thank each and every one of you for allowing me the privilege of speaking to you," she concluded in her talk. "If even one student throws away the cigarettes, I am forever grateful."

Two important things came out of that talk. The first was that Barb got a large batch of letters from students encouraging her to do more talks.

"I've decided to quit, and to stop people from starting," wrote one boy, Matthew Myers. "Thank you for changing my life."

"I told you that I didn't smoke, but to tell you the truth, I have been for a while now," wrote a girl, Courtney Burlet. "But yesterday I took your advice and threw them out!"

Karen Gaudin wrote: "My whole family smokes, so it's been an emotional time, and also for many other of my friends. . . Hopefully what you said will stay in their minds. And just between us girls, you're a knockout, even without your hair."

And from a student with initials P.K.: "If there is anything I want this Christmas, I know on top of my wish list would be for you to live a long life, for a miracle. I would just like to thank you for making me feel life is worth living."

The second important thing was that Tracy had again sent out a call to the news media to cover Barb's talk, and this time, along with reporter Cathy Lord, the *Journal* assigned photographer Greg Southam.

Greg is a veteran and award-winning photographer and a friend of mine. We'd covered many stories together, from sporting events to mass murders, and

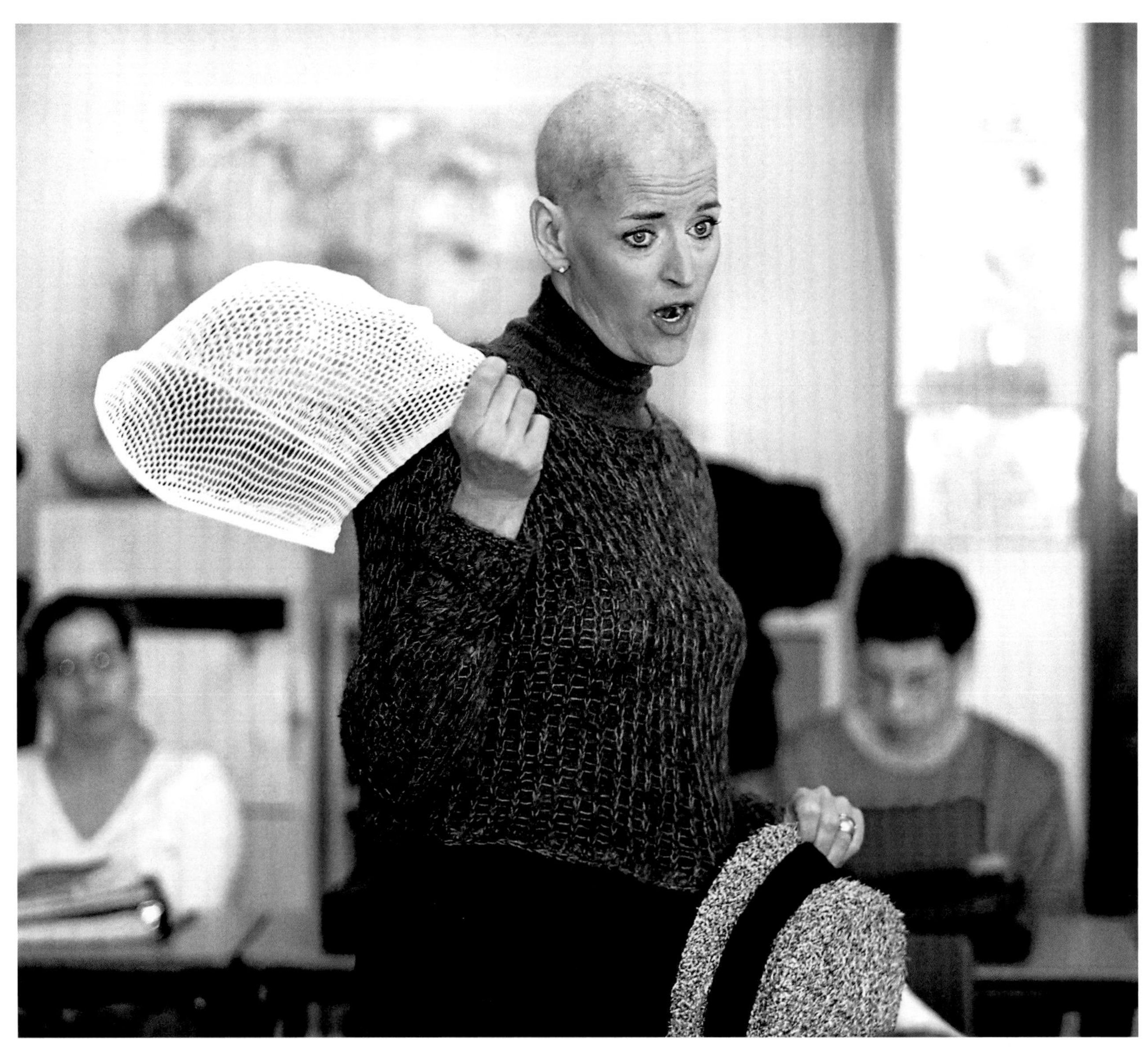

Barb's first presentation was to students at T. D. Baker school on October 29, 2002.

knew each other socially, becoming particularly close in recent years as we both went through the break-ups of long-term relationships.

Barb's talk had moved Greg, but as soon as she was done, he was on to the next job in a busy day, rushing to a car dealership for a shoot. The next morning, however, Greg fell sick with a sore throat. He stayed home from work and, with a moment to slow down, found he was constantly thinking back to Barb and her talk, to how the students had been weeping, as well as all of the media, including himself. Barb's ability to get through to others was astonishing, he thought, as was her willingness to expose herself. Greg realized he had the opportunity to do something more, to see if he could follow her to check ups, to treatments, right to her death bed, in order to show how bad lung cancer really was.

He picked up the phone and dialed Barb's number. When she answered, his tongue felt heavy, mainly because he didn't expect Barb to agree to what he was asking. If he himself were dying, Greg doubted he'd agree to have a photographer around for any personal or unpleasant moments.

Greg explained his plan to Barb, making sure to tell her it wouldn't be easy to have a photojournalist around all the time. Barb cut him off in mid-sentence; Greg was sure that she wasn't interested. Instead, she said: "Let's do it!"

Greg started in, and was glad to see he had a willing subject in Barb. Even when she was smoking, something she might well be sensitive about, she didn't say a word when Greg took her picture.

Greg realized a writer was needed for the project. I was interested at once. Cancer had killed my grandmother, and was just then destroying my uncle, who had also been a long-time smoker. I was haunted, too, by a childhood memory of a hometown neighbor, Robert Doig, a lifelong smoker, coming home from the hospital to visit for the last time, impossibly thin and white-skinned, a cancer-ridden ghost. I wanted to know the ways and means of cancer, how it spreads, how it kills.

In my initial research, I found all the major public health organizations said the same thing: half of all regular smokers eventually die from their habit, either from lung cancer, heart disease, circulatory problems, or a host of other problems directly attributable to smoking. Most of these deaths are premature. Researchers estimate that, on average, smokers lose about 15 years of their lives. In total, smoking causes about 45,000 deaths a year in Canada. The statistics are equally grim in the United States, where the Centers for Disease Control estimates that tobacco causes more than 440,000 deaths each year.

Barb's campaign built up momentum just as Greg started to photograph her. In early November, at a second talk to T.D. Baker students, this time in the large school gym, the Alberta Lung Association sent a cameraman to record the speech for future use in Alberta classrooms. They were keen about Barb, mainly because she was reaching teenagers. Statistics showed that eighty per cent of smokers started when they were teens, one third of them before the age of 15.

Through November, Barb spoke at a handful of other schools and made her first appearance on a popular open-line show hosted by Al Stafford on CHED radio. Stafford was at once taken with how dynamic she was, but he also found himself doubting that she had cancer at all. There had been a recent case in the United States where a woman had lied about having the disease and had collected sympathy as well as a lot money before her deception was revealed.

On the show, Barb faced her first major public relations setback, a caller criticizing her because she was still smoking. At first, she was so upset she wanted to quit doing her talks, but her husband Pat calmed her.

"A lot of the people that are saying that negative stuff are adults, and who cares?" he told her. "You're not after the adults. You're after the kids. The adults have already been smoking for 20 years. They're going to find 20 reasons under the sun not to quit. They'll go on about how this Barb girl still smokes. They'll find excuses for everything."

The notion that Barb was a hypocrite was much on my mind at our first meeting. I felt her mixture of smoking and preaching was dubious. When I asked her about it, she recounted to me how Dr. Halperin had told her that quitting smoking would do her no good. Still, she said, she hated her ongoing addiction and had cut down to five cigarettes a day. "It's sickening. Look at the power of the cigarette! I get very mad. Sometimes, I throw it away."

The only time she had ever been able to quit smoking, she said, was when she was pregnant.

Part of me still wished her crusade was untainted by her smoking, but I accepted her explanation.

Barb was now taking 18 pills a day, some to keep down the swelling around the tumour in her brain, some for pain, some for mouth sores.

She hadn't had a headache in years, she said, but now when she bent over, it felt like her head was going to explode. In her ears, she would sometimes hear the rushing of a train.

To stay upbeat, she named her tumours, calling them Betty Lou. She had stern talks with them where she ordered them to shrink.

Barb did get down when she thought of Mackenzie, and how her daughter had done nothing to deserve being motherless, but it was going to happen anyway. "I'm mad at me. This is my responsibility. I smoked. It was my fault."

Barb's plan was to stay out of the hospital as long as she could, but not too long. She didn't want to die at home, like Michael had. That would be too much for Pat and Mackenzie, she said.

In order to look presentable, Barb wore thick stage make-up. It took her an hour every morning to put it on. She wanted to cover the black beneath her eyes. She lathered on moisturizer because she was so dry and going crazy with itch. She put it all over her head, then put on her foundation, lipstick, eyeliner, mascara. She had taken to wearing a tuque to bed because her head was so cold.

She told Greg that she was going to let him photograph her without the make-up.

"People have to see what happens," she said. "When you say 'lung cancer,' how many people really know what it means to have the disease? It's eating everything inside me. Greg, I want you in there until the very last moment."

"I'll be there," Greg said.

Barb looked back at me. "I am grateful to Greg... I told him, 'It's going to get really bad, and I want the

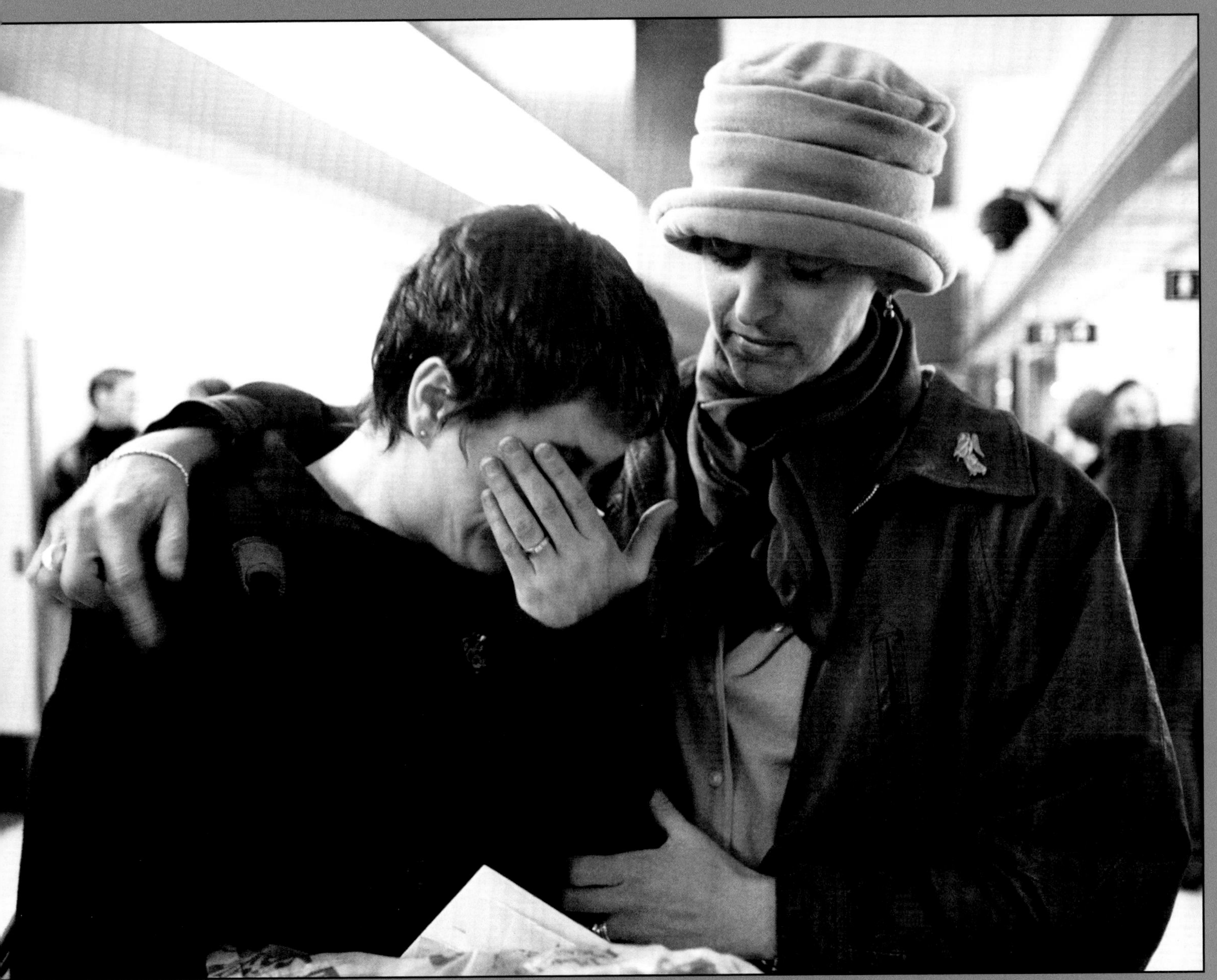

Barb says goodbye to her cousin Carole who is flying home to England knowing they will never see each other again.

ugliest pictures possible, because it's honesty.' People need to see this. I don't want anybody, anybody, walking this path."

What did she think about dying?

"I dread it. I'm leaving my husband and my daughter. I'm leaving my closest friends. There is nothing worse."

What was it like to still be alive?

"I get up every morning and I think, 'God, I am so lucky.' But at the same time I want to stay as long as I can. So every morning when I wake up, I'm grateful, and the first thing I say is, 'Thank you,' and the last thing I say at night is, 'Please give me one more day. I don't want to be greedy, but please, give me one more month.'

"I really have to get through December," Barb continued. "Pat's dad died December 5th. Our son Michael died December 23rd and our son Patrick died December 28th."

As Barb described the circumstances of Michael's death, her emotions rose up in her, red pin pricks in her face.

"Nobody should know what that pain is. There is no worse pain. If there was anything that would destroy me, that was it. There were days I couldn't walk."

Did she and Pat get any counseling?

"Pat and I put all our faith in God, and we always did. Obviously God knows why, and we don't know. Our faith got us through it. We asked to be strong every day. But there isn't a day that goes by where you don't think of your children."

With that, Greg and I departed. We said little on the drive back to the *Journal.*

So much death, I thought. How could all that happen to one family, one woman? Her mother, her twins, now her. I couldn't fathom it. Just then, a superstitious side of me came out and I wondered if Barb was somehow cursed, if there wasn't some dark explanation for all that had gone wrong.

Thursday, November 28. Barb had an appointment with her chemotherapist, Dr. Martin Palmer. She invited me along. "He looks exactly like Robert Redford," she said. "You better prepare yourself for that."

I met Barb and Pat at the Cross Cancer Institute. As tall and slender as Barb was, Pat was even taller and thinner, at 6-feet 5-inches, with dark, greying hair, warm brown eyes, an easy smile.

When I had a moment, I asked him what he thought about Greg and me following Barb during her final days. He had no problems at all, he said.

On Barb's lapel, she wore an angel figurine pin. She told me she had worn one since Michael died.

Various companies had been calling her, she said, telling her about their innovative cures for cancer. "That really annoys me. I have to question the kind of person who would do that to a dying person. If they had the cure for Stage IV, I think I'd know about it."

"People would be beating down the door," Pat said.

"There was one where they wanted me to take 400 pills a day!"

Just then, a nurse came by. "I've seen you in the papers," she said. "You're a very good role model."

"Not really," Barb said. "Not when I smoke."

The nurse asked Barb to fill out a form. Barb checked off her symptoms: difficulty sleeping, pain, tiredness, changes to skin, mouth sores, changes in appetite, nausea, diarrhea, difficulty urinating, changes in sexuality. On the hospital scale, she found she'd dropped from 158 to 142 pounds in two weeks.

We were ushered into Palmer's office. He soon arrived, and, just as Barb said, he had some resemblance to the slender, handsome actor Redford.

"So how you feeling?" he asked with a slight British accent.

"Oh, crap," said Barb.

"I'm not surprised. The inevitable conclusion is that these brain metastases will be getting even bigger now."

"I hate what this is doing to me," Barb said. "I hate it. Is the cancer just this pissed off and aggressive inside my body that there's nothing I can do?"

"Yes, that's the way it is."

As much as she distrusted the miracle cures of the faith healers and homeopaths, Barb still ran them by Palmer. "So I can just ignore all this?"

"When conventional medicine does not have the answers, and in this case it certainly does not, then people are desperate. Many will want to look around for other answers. When people are desperate, their bullshit detector doesn't work so well. This is why alternative treatment is a multi-billion dollar industry."

"They've got nothing to lose," Pat said.

"What they have to lose is money, their savings. This may not affect them, but it can put their family in a very desperate situation. We're obliged to give you the straight goods, as gently as possible, but the problem with the straight goods is, it doesn't give a lot of hope."

"What experimental drugs do you have, and you just need somebody to try?" Barb asked.

"There are currently no drugs for brain metastases," Palmer said. He added that experimental drugs often make it worse for a patient. As for chemotherapy, it might shrink her lung tumours, but it wouldn't get rid of them.

Pat nodded his head. "It'd be like fixing a flat when the engine is the problem."

Barb told Palmer about her fear that she might have a seizure and drop dead in front of a gym full of kids during a presentation.

Before such a seizure, Palmer told her, she would likely feel an aura, and she would be able to take action. Even so, he said, she shouldn't worry. "For those kids you're talking to, if they see that, it would send a powerful message. What you're doing in talking to school kids, I really respect, and I thank you for it. I think it's a profoundly courageous thing to do. This would be a relatively uncommon illness if not for smoking."

Palmer offered to write her a prescription for morphine to control her pain.

"I still think you look like Robert Redford," Barb said in parting.

"Well, shucks," the doctor smiled. "You're about the only person who thought that. How much do I have to pay you for that?"

Outside the office, Barb thought about the doctor's offer of morphine. "I was always one who said I didn't need drugs. I don't even need a Tylenol. But things change."

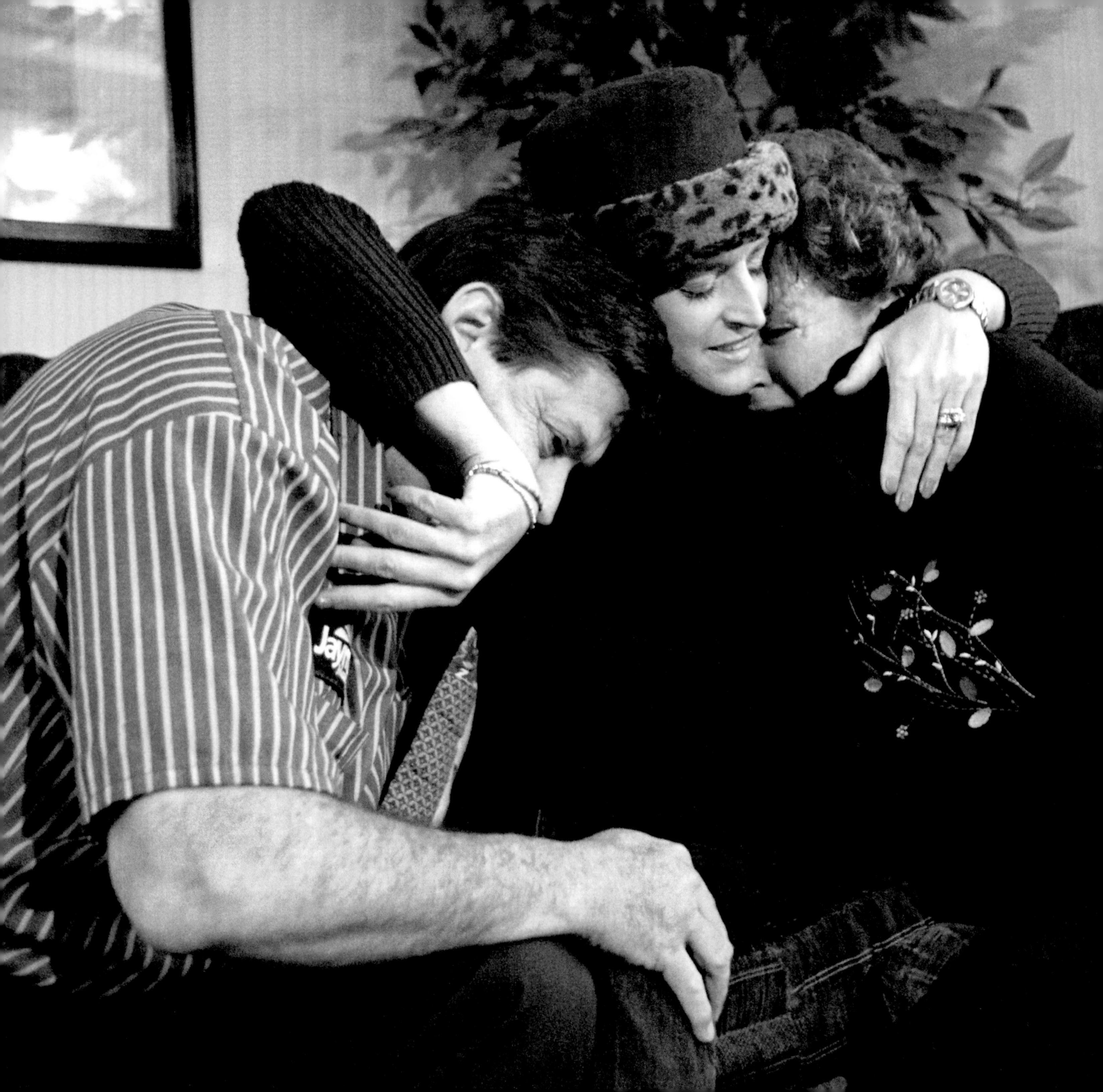

December

2 0 0 2

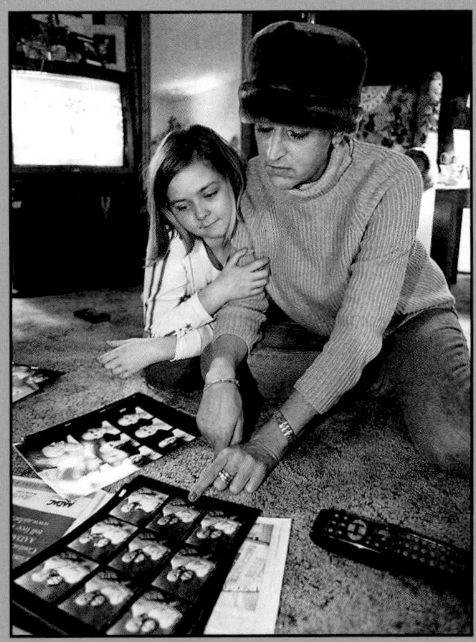

. . . come celebrate
with me that every day
something has tried to kill
me and has failed.

Lucille Clifton

Opposite page: Barb hugs Gary and Adrianna Harris after visiting with them in their home. Gary quit smoking after seeing Barb on television. He had smoked for more than 30 years.

Tuesday, December 3. When I showed up at J. Percy Page High School to hear Barb speak, Barb's friend Tracy was taping posters to the gym wall, one showing the location of Barb's tumours, another with photographs of Barb and Mackenzie cutting off Barb's hair and placing it in trees for the birds.

The students tromped in, flopping down on the gym floor, all chattering.

"This woman, she's dying from cancer," a teacher said to one noisy group. "So could you please pretend to listen."

Barb started out by telling the kids she'd been watching them come into the gym. "I just want to tell you, you guys have great hair!"

She used to work as a fashion model, she said, and used to have wonderful hair herself. Just then, she yanked off her cap to reveal her bald head. "This is what smoking got me, guys!" she said. "After 41 years of hair, I lost mine in 10 days. How cool is it? You know what? I don't think it's cool at all.

"Why did I smoke?" she continued. "Because I wanted to be in the 'in' crowd. They were all so popular. Yeah, they were getting into mischief, but they were hanging out, they were going to parties, they were doing the things I thought were the coolest."

Barb passed around the plastic mask from her radiation treatment. Every student touched it.

"This is reality!" she told them. "You smoke, this is what happens!"

Barb spoke about the link between smoking and cancer as if it were a certainty for every smoker, which, of course, it is not. The majority of smokers will not get lung cancer, though one in 19 women and two in 23 men in Canada will be hit by the lethal disease in their lifetime. In 85 per cent of those cases, smoking is the culprit.

Barb listed some of the foul chemicals in cigarettes to the students. "Why don't you just smoke your toilet bowl cleaner? Because that's what's in a cigarette!"

Vivid descriptions, such as this toilet bowl cleaner metaphor, peppered Barb's speech, but the thing that most impressed me was her ability to tell a story.

She'd been shopping at a store just before Halloween, she said, and a five-year-old had looked at her in her hat and thick make-up.

"Mommy, someone should tell her Halloween is over," the child said.

Recalling those words, Barb shook her head and moaned softly. "Oh, oh, oh, oh, how do you think I felt?" She paused, looked down. "Pain," she whispered. "I felt sorry for myself."

Every teen was focused on her now. She stared into their eyes. "Look how cool I am, guys. Look at me! *Look at me!*"

They all wept. The teachers wept. Greg and Tracy wept, and I wept, too, moved by Barb's force and her fragility. She was like a glorious bouquet, an explosion of colour and life, but cut at the stem, soon to die.

I was no smoker, but when she talked of Mackenzie growing up without a mother, she made me think of my own mortality and of my own three sons, one of them born within a month of Mackenzie. I knew how much they needed me, and what a loss my death would be for them.

There was, however, one jarring note for me in Barb's talk. I'd always found people to be much more relaxed and open in private than on stage, but not Barb. She said exactly the same things in the same way

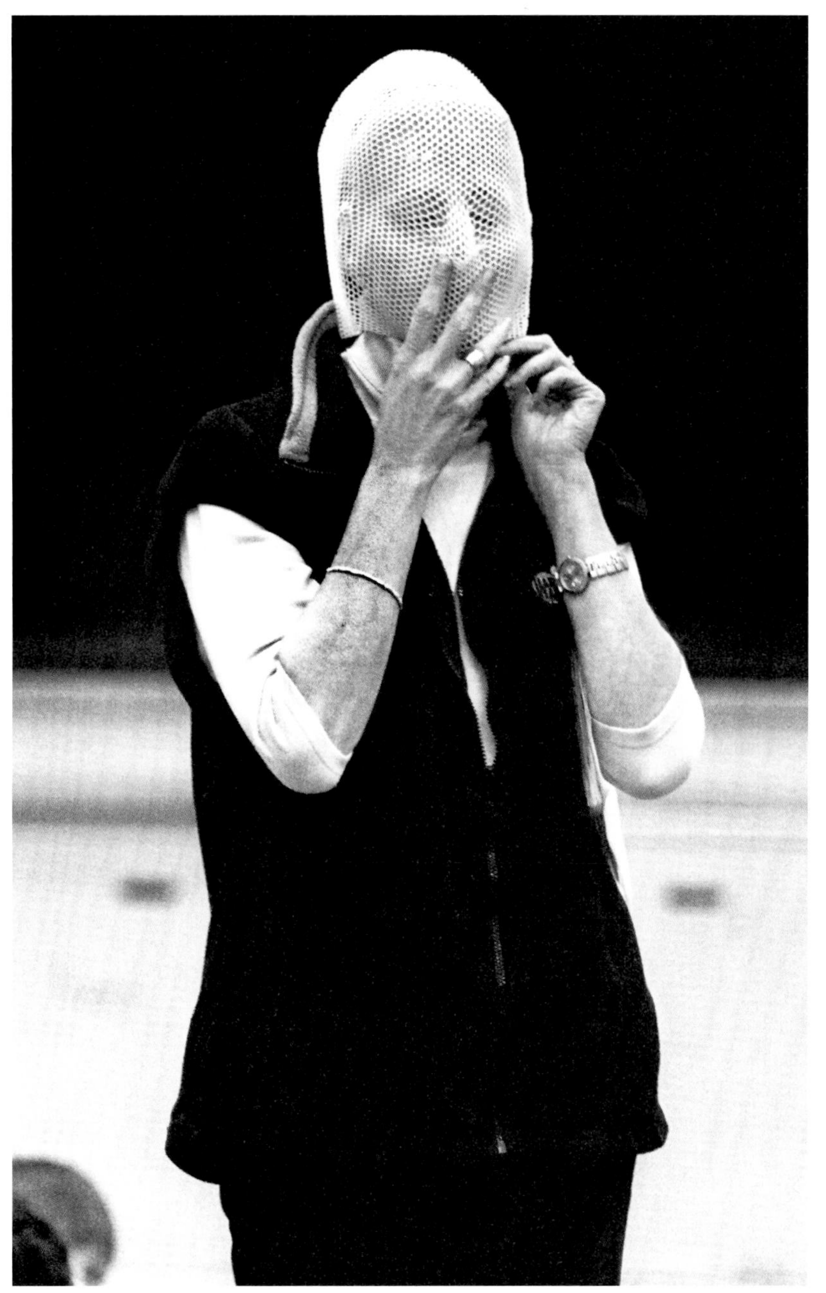

Barb talks to students at Holy Cross school about what it is like to receive radiation as she shows them the mask she wore during the treatment.

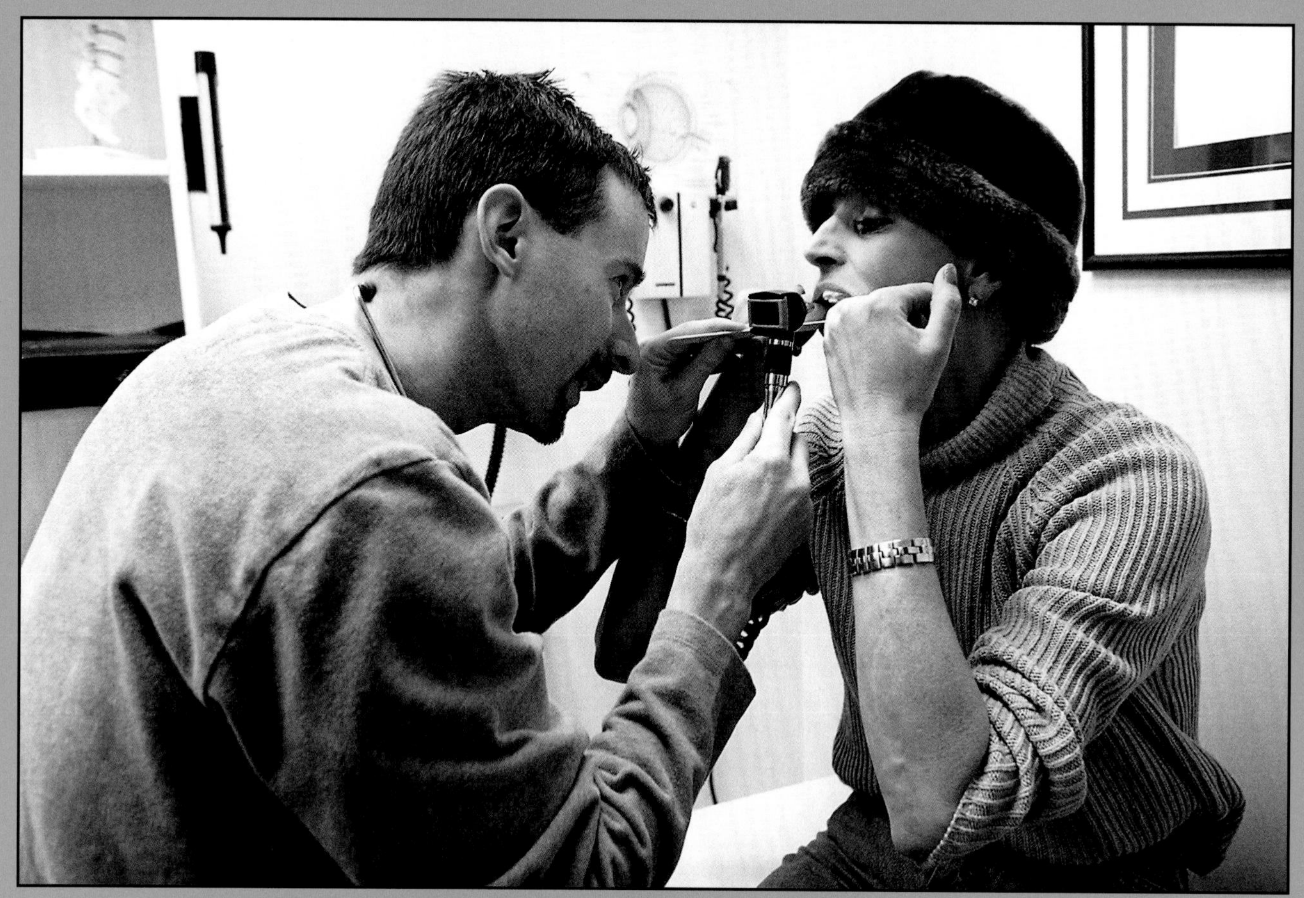

Dr. Douglas Fonteyne checks Barb's mouth after she mentions she has many sores that are bothering her.

to the students as she had said to me in our interview. This reminded me of a clever politician, always sticking to the message, revealing not one thing more in private than to the crowd.

Or maybe, I thought, Barb always spoke from the heart, so there was no need to ever alter her message. I didn't know.

Afterwards, a mob of kids surrounded her. She looked at them with adoring eyes, admired their hair, and held their hands.

"Oh, you're so nice and warm," she said.

Wednesday, December 4. Barb spoke to a large group of high school students at Fort High in Fort Saskatchewan. Principal Eleanore Commodore wrote Barb and described how the school had been during the talk: "We have 535 students and 40 staff and the only noise you could hear was tears hitting the floor."

Thursday, December 5. On the way to see Barb's family physician, Barb told Tracy about all the Christmas shopping she'd done for Mackenzie.

"I just want to give her her every dream."

"What she wants, you can't give," Tracy said.

Barb was quiet for a moment. "I know," she said.

Tracy pulled up and stopped in front of the main door of the Mill Woods building where Dr. Douglas Fonteyne had his office.

"You want me to drop you off at the door, then I'll go park?" Tracy asked.

"You want me to smack you!" Barb fired back, determined not to be treated as an invalid.

Barb checked her make-up in the car mirror

"This is the best you've ever looked," Tracy told her.

"You just like the bald look," Barb said.

I could see Barb and Tracy had a good friendship, one that allowed for a healthy amount of ribbing. They both loved to laugh and poke fun and Barb's cancer wasn't going to stop them.

Dr. Douglas Fonteyne was a young man, obviously smart, with a friendly, laid-back bedside manner. Barb sat on a raised bed as he examined her.

"You know what?" she said. "It's a mess, the headaches, the pain."

"Are you taking anything for it right now?"

"Yes, I'm taking the pills right now."

"How much of the Tylenol are you taking?"

"One a day."

Fonteyne urged her to take Tylenol 3 and to consider going on morphine. "I wouldn't suffer with it," he said of her condition. "The last thing you want to do is put up with a headache."

Barb said she was having no bowel movements, and that she wasn't sleeping well at all. Fonteyne asked if she had thought about palliative care.

"I want to stay preferably at home two days before I go into a coma," she said. "And then put me in the Grey Nuns."

"Are you sure you don't want to die at home?"

"I can't, Dr. Fonteyne. I just don't want to die at home."

He checked Barb's blood pressure, her breathing.

"Is there any sign that might come that will tell me when it's coming?" she asked of her impending collapse.

"No," Fonteyne said, shaking his head. "Only He knows."

He ended the check-up by repeating that Barb

should think about pain relief. Two tablets of morphine a day might make a huge difference. "You don't get any points for suffering."

Barb just nodded, but didn't agree. She said she feared the drugs might make her too sluggish to speak to the kids.

"Just get some rest," Fonteyne said. "Any kids you can turn off cigarettes, that's good. Keep going. Just get some rest."

Saturday, December 7. After her talk in Fort Saskatchewan, the students decided each one should write her a letter saying what her presentation had meant to them. Students then found Barb's address in Mill Woods. On Saturday morning, a delegation dropped off a box of letters.

Every single non-smoking student said they had been convinced to never smoke, but Barb was most moved by the 60 students who smoked and promised to quit.

"I am just at the start of my fourth year of smoking and am on the verge of quitting, but to do that is just killing me," wrote one, Joe Fertuck. "I have tried to stop. I cough. I have sore throats, but the addiction that is in me overcomes my well-being. I generally assumed when I started that I could quit when I wanted, but, no, it doesn't work like that. Sometimes, I swear I ask my mom to lock me up for days, weeks, to make me stop. I can't run. I can't play hockey like I love to because I am short of breath. . . I am happy you have made the choice to come to our school and talk to us in the manner you have chosen, very straightforward, cause that is the only way the point will ever reach somebody as myself."

Wednesday, December 11. On the way to Barb's speaking engagement in Spruce Grove, a town just outside of Edmonton, Barb turned to Tracy, who, as usual, was driving.

"It's gonna be soon," Barb said.

"What?"

"My death. It's gonna be soon."

Tracy wasn't sure what to think. Barb certainly wasn't eating much. On the other hand, her desire to smoke was as strong as ever. During the 30-minute drive that morning, she'd chain-smoked four cigarettes. Tracy asked her why she was smoking so much again.

"I don't know what's wrong with me," Barb said, but went to light up another one.

"Barb, you don't need another."

"Just let me," Barb said, thrusting the cigarette in her mouth. "Just let me."

I met the two in the lobby of St. Marguerite Catholic School, a junior high. Barb looked more frail today, her skin dry and shriveled. She had been trying to eat oranges and a nutritional drink, but without much luck. "Whooey, did I throw up!" she said and laughed.

Barb had also been experiencing memory loss. She had been smoking in her car, she said, and went to put out her cigarette, only to stick the burning cigarette into her purse.

The school had a huge sign up on the gym wall: "Welcome Barb Tarbox."

Barb began her talk. In a few short days, I noticed her performance had grown in its power. It was more nuanced now, more theatrical, her face contorting into ever more obvious emotions: sadness, anger, disdain, acceptance. She waved her arms in ever wider arcs to make her points.

She told the students that her latest symptom was white goo coming out of her mouth, nose and eyes, then painted a gruesome picture of her experience with radiation therapy. "Let me tell you what the cigarette does. It *burns you*! Radiation *fries* your brain. It puts a hole in your brain."

I ducked into the hallway to interview Tracy about her relationship with Barb.

She told me she was pleased to see the vitriol coming out of Barb. "She's just amazing! I think it's rage we're seeing. She's in the angry stage, and it all comes out when she's speaking to the kids. This is perfect for her to be doing. I think this is keeping her alive. She wakes up in the morning looking forward to this."

She and Barb first got to know each other through their daughters of the same age, Miranda and Mackenzie, who went to the same school, Tracy said. She had met Barb about five years back while volunteering at a school hot dog stand.

Tracy was attracted to Barb's outgoing nature. Both of them were smokers as well, though Tracy only smoked when she was out with friends, not at home, or at work. "I'm only smoking with Barb until her death," she said. "She's made me promise, and I gave her my guarantee."

Most often, the two would have a smoke before Barb went in for her presentations, Tracy said. She made sure to spritz Barb with perfume so no one would smell cigarettes on her.

She and Barb had never been the kind of friends who went out and socialized all the time, Tracy said, partly because Barb mostly stayed at home. Until recently, Tracy hadn't even known that Barb was married; Pat was never around in the evenings. When she finally did meet Pat, Tracy teased him that he was Barb's rent-a-husband.

Barb and Tracy had become close friends in 1999, after the death of Michael. Afterwards, Barb got a lovely card in the shape of an angel from a woman who said she'd read about Michael's death in the newspaper and wanted to offer her sympathy and support, partly because she had lost her own son.

"Is that woman's name Jane?" Tracy had asked.

"Yes," Barb said. "How did you know?"

Tracy told Barb that Jane was her mother, Jane Orydzuk, and that ever since her son (and Tracy's brother) Tim had been killed in a strange and still unsolved murder case in 1993, Jane had been going through the newspaper obits and sending out cards to other grieving parents.

Tracy, too, had been devastated by Tim's death. In Barb, she found someone else who knew what it truly meant to suffer. She had never before had such a friend.

"I don't know how we feel so connected, but we're connected," Tracy said.

The two often talked about the afterlife, how Tracy might one day talk to Tim, and about how Barb would see her twins. In recent weeks, Tracy said, Barb no longer seemed so sad about saying good-bye to Mackenzie. "Either she's got really used to the idea of dying, or she's very excited to see Patrick and Michael again. She's got her things to look forward to on the other side. She'll see her kids again. And she's very excited about seeing my brother."

Barb told Tracy that after she was gone, she was

going to be reincarnated as a butterfly, and would come back to watch over Tracy. Butterflies were of special significance to Barb. When little Patrick had died, the nurses had placed a butterfly sticker on Michael's crib, a memorial to his lost brother. Last summer, Barb told Tracy, she had been in her backyard when a butterfly had landed on her and stayed for 20 minutes. Barb believed it to be a message from her boys.

Barb and Tracy liked to watch John Edward, a New York medium who purported to connect people with their deceased loved ones. "Barb told me that next year, if I can get on the show, she'll come through, she'll be there. She also told me she'll help me win the lottery," Tracy said and laughed. "She'll send down the numbers, she said. I said, 'Barb, you're not God.' "

The two also liked to talk about their dreams, and what they might portend for the future. Barb had had a dream two years back about speaking in gyms, with kids, teachers. Tracy was in the gym as well, along with government dignitaries. That might happen soon, Tracy said. It would be a sign that Barb's goal had been accomplished here. "Maybe this was meant to be. I don't know."

Tracy laughed a moment later, aware that she had been saying a lot, but didn't know what I thought about all her beliefs.

I told her I wasn't much of a believer in this kind of thing, not that I had all the answers myself.

Tracy told me her relationship with Barb had really taken off in October, when she had offered to drive Barb to her radiation treatments. From the start, Tracy said she was impressed with Barb's lack of self-pity.

"Barb never, ever said to me, 'Why is this happening to me?' Never once."

It was good that more and more schools wanted Barb, Tracy said, but she admitted the crusade was also becoming a strain. She was waking up in the middle of the night, thinking about Barb and all that needed to be done.

"I'm a basketcase. I'm like my mother. When somebody needs somebody, I'm just there, totally 100-per-cent committed. I feel like I can't say, 'No.' I don't want to deny Barb anything in the last weeks of life, and I hope I would have a friend who would do this for me if I was dying. I don't want to say, 'No.' And I'm so glad to be part of this. I'm so honoured. But this is Barb's life. I have another life. I'm struggling to get everything done."

A few weeks back, Tracy had had to sit down with her bosses at Team Ford and tell them if they had to replace her, she would understand that, but she needed time for Barb. Her bosses had scoffed at her offer to resign, and told Tracy to do her duty to Barb. Even with their blessing, Tracy felt guilty about work. Every day, 20 or 30 calls came in related to Barb, from schools, media, well-wishers. Then there were all the presentations to attend. Tracy knew if she refused to take Barb, Barb would just cancel. But Tracy's real work was piling up. After a full day of travel with Barb, she had started working nights at Team Ford. "I don't tell Barb that because she feels bad."

The one thing she was starting to resent, Tracy said, was that Pat had yet to come see Barb talk, and didn't appear to be keen to drive her to any presentations either. Barb was also still carrying a full load at home, Tracy said, doing all the shopping and cleaning, paying the bills. She wished Pat would do more. She also wanted to limit the number of Barb's out-of-town talks, have her concentrate on Edmonton schools. "I feel sorry for the smokers. I want them to quit as much as Barb does. I don't want anybody to end up like Barb. But I don't know if I'd spend the end of my life doing this for somebody else. That's where I'm totally opposite to Barb. I don't think I'd wallow in self-pity because I'm strong. But I don't think I'd be doing this. But Barb says this gives her strength. When we're driving to these things, she's so excited, it's like insane."

Just then, we noticed that Barb's talk had ended. A group of girls now enveloped her in a massive, weeping hug. Barb smiled, looked into their eyes, admired their unblemished skin, shining hair and eyes.

"Oh, look at all the hair," she said. "I'm so jealous of you guys. You guys are magic."

"My parents smoke and I don't want them to die," one little girl told Barb.

"Sometime you just go talk to Mom," Barb told her. "Hold her, hold her hand, and say, 'I love you with all my heart and can we talk about this and what we can do together?' Let's say, 'Mom, instead of having another cup of coffee and a cigarette, let's go walking in the mall or let's go swimming.' That helps change the habit."

Off to the side, principal Steve Dempsey admired Barb's work. "I've never seen anyone touch kids like her."

On her way out, Barb got a hug from Tony McDonald, a staff member and a smoker for 40 years. He was weeping.

"God bless you," Barb said, then spoke quietly with the man. He nodded, wept some more, wiped tears from his eyes and wished her well.

"Boy, I'll tell you, I think we just increased the stock of Kleenex," Dempsey said.

Later in the afternoon, Barb called me up to say that Calder Bateman, the advertising firm handling the account for the provincial government's anti-smoking agency, the Alberta Alcohol and Drug Addiction Commission (AADAC), had called her to say it wanted to use her for a TV campaign.

"This is just getting stranger!" Barb crowed. "This is insane!"

AADAC also wanted Barb to speak at a school in Calgary, to spread her message to another major market.

Was she healthy enough for such a trip, I asked?

The pain was worse than ever, she said, but whenever she felt too much she now thought about her son. "Michael taught me never to quit, never give up, no matter what obstacle you have. The pain, I can still bear more. Michael taught me well."

Saturday, December 14. For the first time, Barb took morphine.

Monday, December 16. With Barb speaking in Calgary on Thursday, and with AADAC taking her on as a spokesperson, her crusade had reached a new level, which pushed me to do a news story in the *Journal* on newfound success. I phoned her radiologist, Dr. Halperin.

"Barb is sacrificing some of her remaining good hours for the betterment of her community and I can't think of many things more noble," Halperin said. "I hope that when my time comes to answer the bell, that I answer it as well as Barbara."

Later, I called Barb to tell her what Halperin had said.

For a moment, she was silent.

"That's good," she said at last, choked up. "That puts colour in my face. You know what? I don't have half the strength today because I'm not talking to these kids today. I'm giving to the community, but what I get back is 1,000 times. They're going to have full lives and they will never smoke."

She told me she had been feeling so poorly that she had cancelled two out-of-town trips. Still, she was prepared for Calgary on Wednesday.

"Wait until you see me Wednesday. I got things up my sleeve, baby."

She was on and off the morphine tablets, she said. "I hate it. I don't like it. But I respect it, and I respect what I have to do. But I feel like I'm giving in to the cancer by taking drugs. I know that is stupid, but that's how I feel."

At her check-up later that day, Barb detailed her new problems to Dr. Fonteyne. Her diarrhea was unrelenting. She also had a temporary loss of her vision. A few times, she'd fallen down as she tried to walk. Once, she had to stay down for five minutes before regaining feeling in her legs. She also brought up her memory loss, how she would write things down on a notepad so she wouldn't forget them, but would then lose the notepad.

"We could tack it to you," Fonteyne suggested.

"God, I'm ready to carve it into my skin."

Barb told the doctor she had booked two final schools, but then would be off until January 7. After that, however, she was going to book and book and

Barb watches an AADAC public service announcement for the first time after taping the ad.

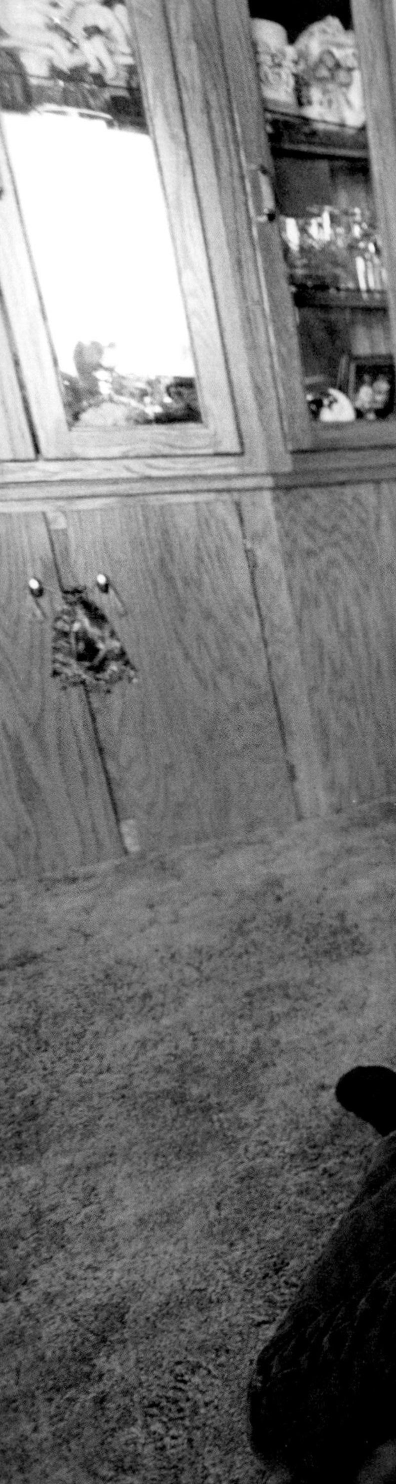

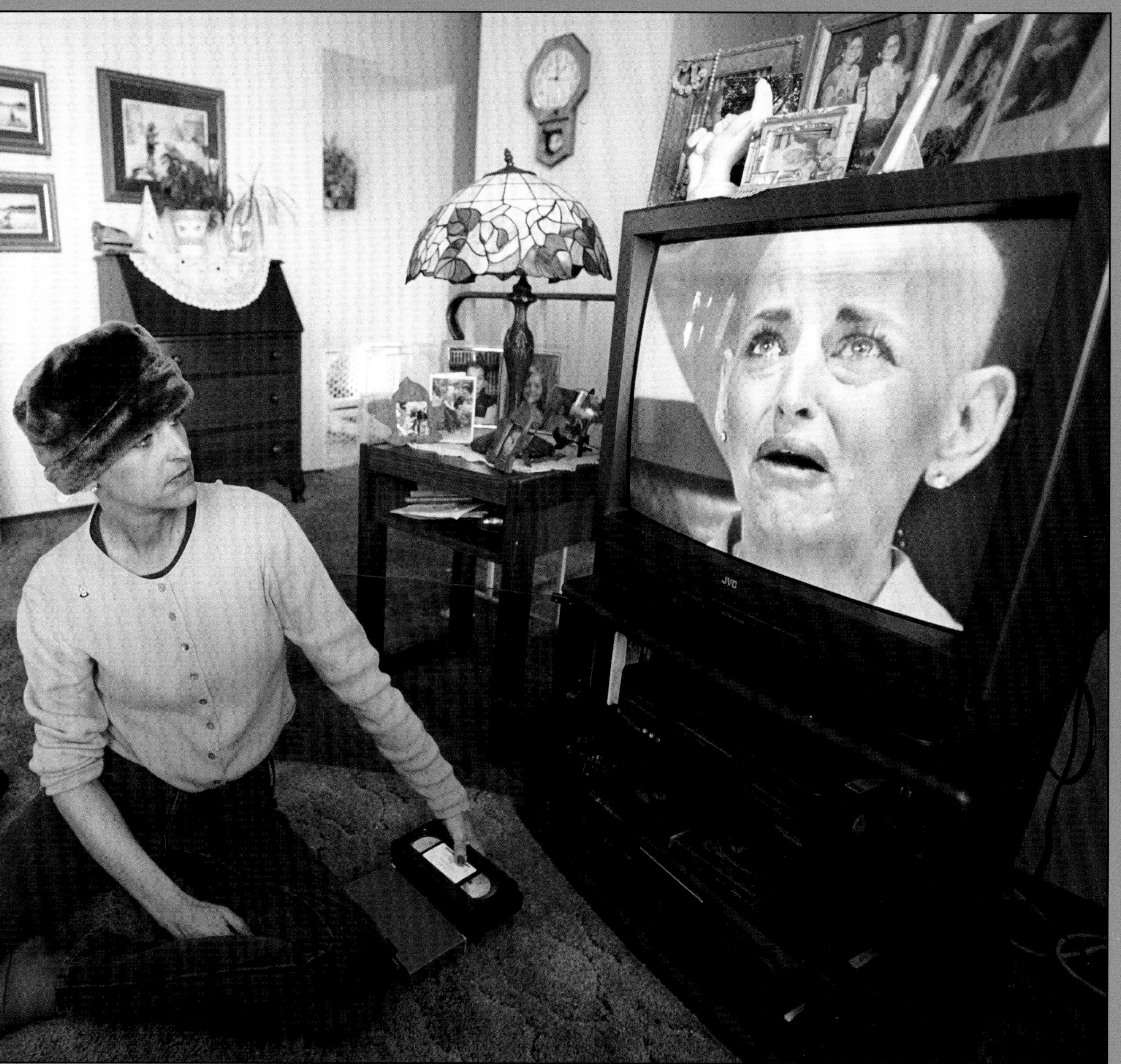
JVC

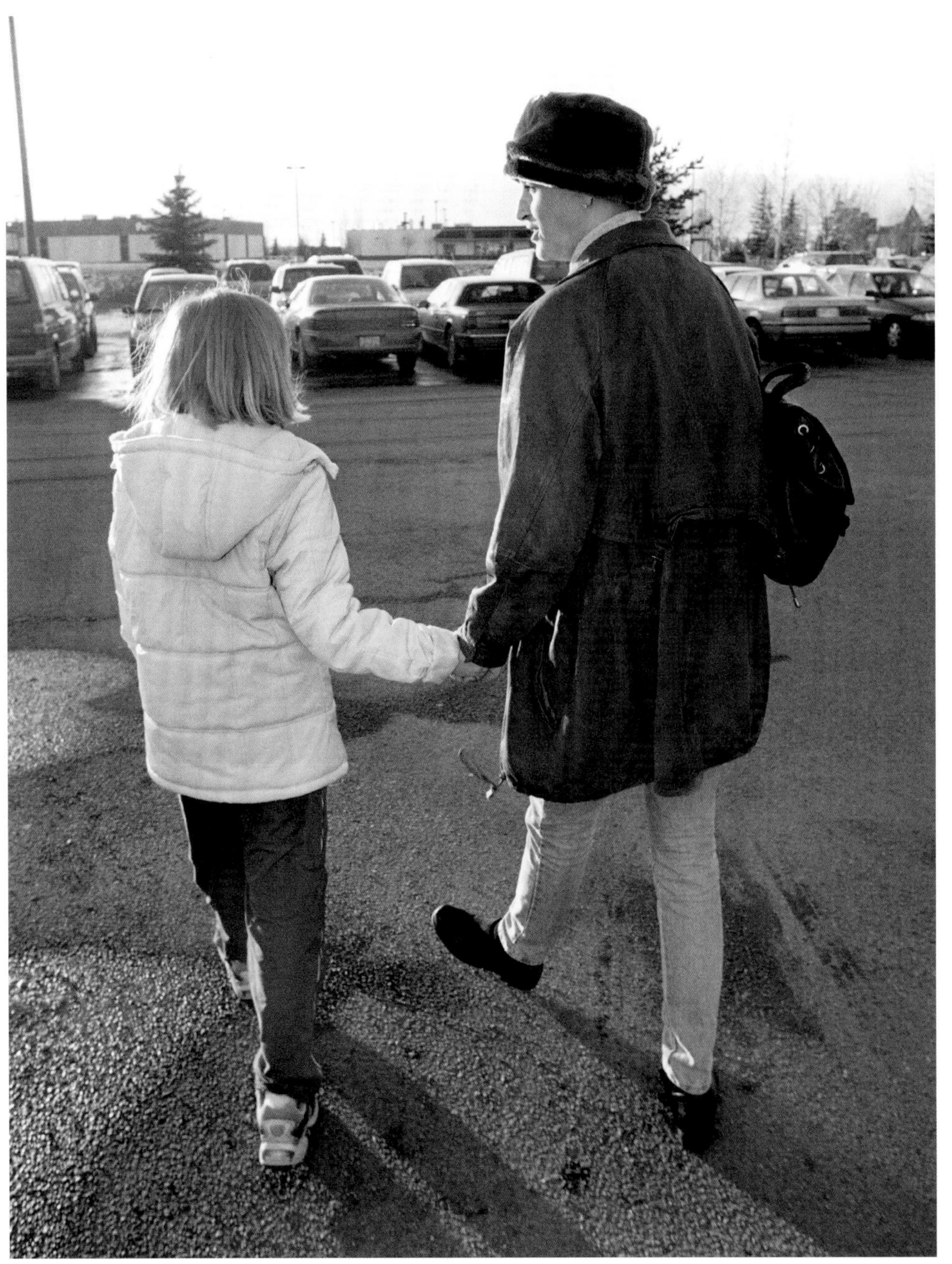

Barb and Mackenzie leave Dr. Fonteyne's office on their way to pick up some KFC for supper.

book. "I'm going to really irritate Betty Lou, my many Betty Lous, by booking through January."

After we left the office, I asked Barb which song she had got 'Betty Lou' from.

"You know, the old Buddy Holly song," she replied.

I paused for a moment, searched my memory. I figured I knew her well enough by now to gently correct her on this point. "You know, I think that song was 'Peggy Sue,' "

Barb looked glum for a moment.

"I don't like that song," she said.

Just then, she brightened up. "No wonder she hasn't been co-operating with me! I've been calling her the wrong name."

Tuesday, December 17. Al Stafford from CHED sent Barb a note, telling her about a truck driver who heard her on the open-line show: "He's been smoking for 25 years. He has two children, aged three and four. He told me to tell you he is praying for you, and you saved his life. And he was in tears. He hasn't smoked in 10 days. Congratulations, Barb!"

In the morning, I sat down to interview Pat at the pub he managed on Bourbon Street at mammoth West Edmonton Mall, the city's major tourist attraction. As Pat described it to me, he and Barb had a traditional relationship. "We agreed to certain responsibilities. She'd be the stay-at-home mom, make sure the kids weren't brought up by babysitters or in daycare."

Pat's job was to bring home the paycheque, even if that meant working two or three jobs at once. He had been in the hospitality business for 25 years, often working extra shifts, six or seven days per week.

"This is my career," he had told Barb when they first started dating. "If it doesn't fit into your scenario, let's end it now, so we won't be miserable six months from now."

Since he had married, he said, he had likely eaten 100 meals at home, as he worked almost every single evening. He had an out-of-town job one year, and was home just 42 days that entire time.

If Barb ever told him that she needed him, Pat said, he would be there in a second. But even when she was caring for Michael, an arduous task, she almost always handled things on her own. "If she wasn't a strong person, I would have had to be home more."

Pat said his strength at work was coming into a new restaurant and whipping things into shape, bringing in order. In fact, he couldn't tolerate it if things were out of place, an attitude that had so far prevailed with Barb's illness as well. It didn't make sense for Mackenzie to quit school, or for him to quit his job so that they could be with Barb all day, he said. Barb could live for another year, he thought, no matter what the doctors said.

"What am I supposed to do? Stop working? That's not how we lived our lives so far, so that's not how we'll live them now. I'm trying to keep things as normal as possible for Mackenzie. I'm really not concerned about me. I'm concerned about Mackenzie."

Pat said he wasn't one to fall apart, especially when his family needed him. When his dad died of a heart attack at 54, he handled funeral arrangements coolly and efficiently, so much so that his sisters had accused him of being heartless and not loving his dad. Pat didn't see it that way. His job wasn't to break down weeping, it was to take care of the family, stand up for everyone, make sure that everything had been handled. He would do the same thing now, he said, and deal with things as they came up.

The media had started to ask questions about why Barb was speaking at schools rather than spending all her time at home with her family.

Pat told me he strongly supported what Barb was doing. And most often, he said, Barb was speaking during the day when he was at work and Mackenzie was at school, so she wasn't missing time with them. Most of all, the speaking was keeping Barb alive, he said. "I think it's great. This is unlike normal cancer patients who are dying, who usually just spend time with their families. It's commendable. It gives her fire. It gives her a reason to get up and keep going.

"Nobody understands this," he continued. "Who is this lady? Why is she doing it? She speaks straight from the heart. Everyone hears all the stats and numbers, but they mean nothing compared to someone standing in front of you who is alive and who is now dying. This cancer now has a name."

His only concern was Barb's stamina. "I've told her to slow down for herself, for me and Mackenzie: 'You have to learn to say No.' She just feels pressed for time. But it's what Barb wants to do. So why would I want to stop her? It wouldn't be fair to her, and it wouldn't be fair to the other smokers. With the media, I'm sharing Barb and my family with millions of people, and that's OK, if people become more health conscious."

As our talk wound down, we chatted about Barb's continued smoking.

Pat said he wasn't surprised that she had kept at it because she'd never been able to quit. He had pushed her a few times, but she was never open to it.

I mentioned to Pat that Barb had, in fact, managed to quit twice before, when she was pregnant.

No, Pat said, that wasn't the case. Barb hadn't quit during either pregnancy, he said, though she had cut down.

After the interview, I thought about Barb's lie. Why do it? Did she blame herself for Patrick and Michael's health problems?

At the office, I researched the effects of smoking on pregnant women. Premature labour is twice as common in pregnant smokers, I found, and there is a higher risk of placental problems. The babies of smokers tend to be smaller, and there is growing evidence they are at greater risk of developmental problems, such as delayed speech, cerebral palsy, visual and hearing difficulties, learning disabilities and respiratory problems. They are also more likely to die in infancy.

It was all damning stuff.

Surely Barb knew the facts about smoking and pregnancy, I thought. Perhaps, though, after Patrick's death, then Michael's disabilities and his death, she was also smart enough and desperate enough to run as fast as she could from her own culpability. It would be far too painful to handle.

I knew I'd have to press her on this issue, but her deception didn't dampen my enthusiasm for her. The core of her message, that smoking kills, was strong, intact and doing a tremendous amount of good. I was sure of that, so much so that I decided to e-mail news of Barb's coming presentation in Calgary to the Alberta correspondents of Canada's two national papers, the *Globe & Mail* and the *National Post*. I knew both reporters well and hoped to sell them on Barb's story so that it might start getting national attention.

I'd never done such a thing before. *No cheering in the press box* is a well-known motto of the craft. With Barb, however, the crusader in me was coming out. I wanted to share her performance with everyone, so that they would be moved in the same way I had been. So I did a little cheering. To hell with press box conventions.

Wednesday, December 18. Barb got up at 2:30 a.m., unable to sleep because of her diarrhea and because she was so excited about the Calgary trip.

Tracy, Barb, Greg and I all went down in a van driven by a young Calder Bateman executive, Craig Marler. He was becoming an integral part of Barb's team, handling many of the details of Barb's AADAC campaign.

The day was cool and clear. Barb appeared to be in good form. She mentioned her misnaming of the tumours. "I feel more strength now that I got the right name, Peggy Sue," she said.

We all laughed.

I worried that we would have to stop every few minutes because of her diarrhea, and maybe never get to Calgary. But Barb never once complained during the three hour trip down Highway 2, though she did ask to stop in Leduc, just outside of Edmonton, so she could have a smoke break.

Tracy, too, had a concern, that Barb wouldn't have the strength to make it through her entire presentation, which usually lasted about 70 to 90 minutes. "Maybe I should get you a stool," Tracy suggested.

"I don't want to sit," Barb said, shaking her head. "The energy from the moment you walk in the school, it just pumps you up. It's incredible. I have enough time to sit on the bed or the couch."

A dozen reporters showed up at Father James Whelihan school, including Bob Remington of the *Post*.

"It's late," she told the kids during her talk. "I'm dying. I have weeks. I have a nurse coming to my house. But I'm not going to let it stop me from telling the most intelligent people that we have what smoking can do. I just flatly refuse to let smoking take another life before its time."

She admitted to the kids that she had tried to get others to smoke when she was a teen, offering them cigarettes. "Why did I do that? To be popular."

By now, Barb's performance had become so polished that sometimes it seemed to me I wasn't watching a dying woman at all, but some marvelous actor. Stomping about, spitting her lines, lashing her arms, wailing, seething, howling, Barb didn't so much as touch the children with her words now as she pummelled them. It was a personal rant, harsh, negative, dark, not like the feel-good puffery of anti-smoking campaigns in the 1990s, which soft-peddled the nasty health effects of smoking and instead tried to build self-esteem in kids so they wouldn't want to smoke. Barb's message was so raw that she never booked an elementary school, believing the kids couldn't take it.

The climax was always Barb pulling off her hat, focusing everything on that bald, cancerous visage. Even if the kids never remembered a word she said, they would be haunted by that spectre. It was perfect for an increasingly visual culture, even one where children were used to seeing horrific images. Barb was the real thing — real skin, real blood, real death. Get close enough to her and you could see the garish make-up, the pallid skin, the gaunt body, the darkness under her eyes.

"Yes, this is gross!" she said. "Yes, it's uncomfortable! Yes, I hate it! This is what smoking does."

Next, Barb pulled out a photograph of her hugging Tracy, one that Greg had taken and had given to her. This was the trick Barb had earlier hinted to me she had up her sleeve.

"This is my best friend Tracy," she said. "And I have to say good-bye to her. The next place she will see me is my funeral."

Barb asked the children to look at a friend and imagine saying good-bye to them. "The thought of not seeing Tracy and my husband and my daughter, it rips my heart apart."

I was sitting next to Tracy, and could see a spasm hit her. She sniffled and wept. I did, too.

"I will never, ever forgive myself for putting them through this," Barb said.

In the question-and-answer session, one of the students asked Barb, "Are you scared?"

"Well, God is with you every day," Barb said. "Now He carries me."

After Barb was done talking, I asked Tracy about the gesture with the photograph.

"Barb won't be doing that again," she said. "That's too hard. That's way too hard. I can't take it."

Of course, Barb didn't agree. It was too moving a gesture to drop. It was also the truth.

On hand was Frank Calder, co-owner of Calder Bateman, who had pushed hard for Barb to be adopted as the spokesperson for AADAC. Calder had hired a camera crew to record the Calgary talk. "The critical thing was to capture it as it was happening," he said. "She's amazing. She's brave, and I think that's what we respond to. Like those little girls getting her autograph. You don't have to be 30 years old to recognize courage."

The strength of Barb's story was its simplicity, Calder said: "She smoked, she's dying, there are people who are left behind who will suffer immensely. It's unvarnished, unembellished and undeniable. If it came from someone else, like a doctor or AADAC, it has some value, but with her, it's there right now, today, and maybe not in another week."

As we were leaving the school, an 11-year-old student, Tanya Marcolin, came up to Barb.

"I hope you're happy in heaven," she said.

On the way home, we stopped at a restaurant. I sat next to Barb. As she ate, I saw the white goo she had previously mentioned at the corner of her mouth. I also caught a whiff of medicine from her, a hospital smell, one I associated with disease. I lost my appetite.

Barb slept most of the way home. Tracy told us a story of a woman who had called, an owner of a motivational speaking company, who wanted to hire Barb as a speaker. "Tell me her name isn't really Tarbox," the woman had said to Tracy.

The woman went on to say that in the old days there were no paper filters on cigarettes, just plastic filters, which gathered up tar, and were then emptied out in a container known as a tarbox.

"Isn't it ironic?" the woman had asked.

Tracy didn't see the humour. She didn't give the woman Barb's number, either.

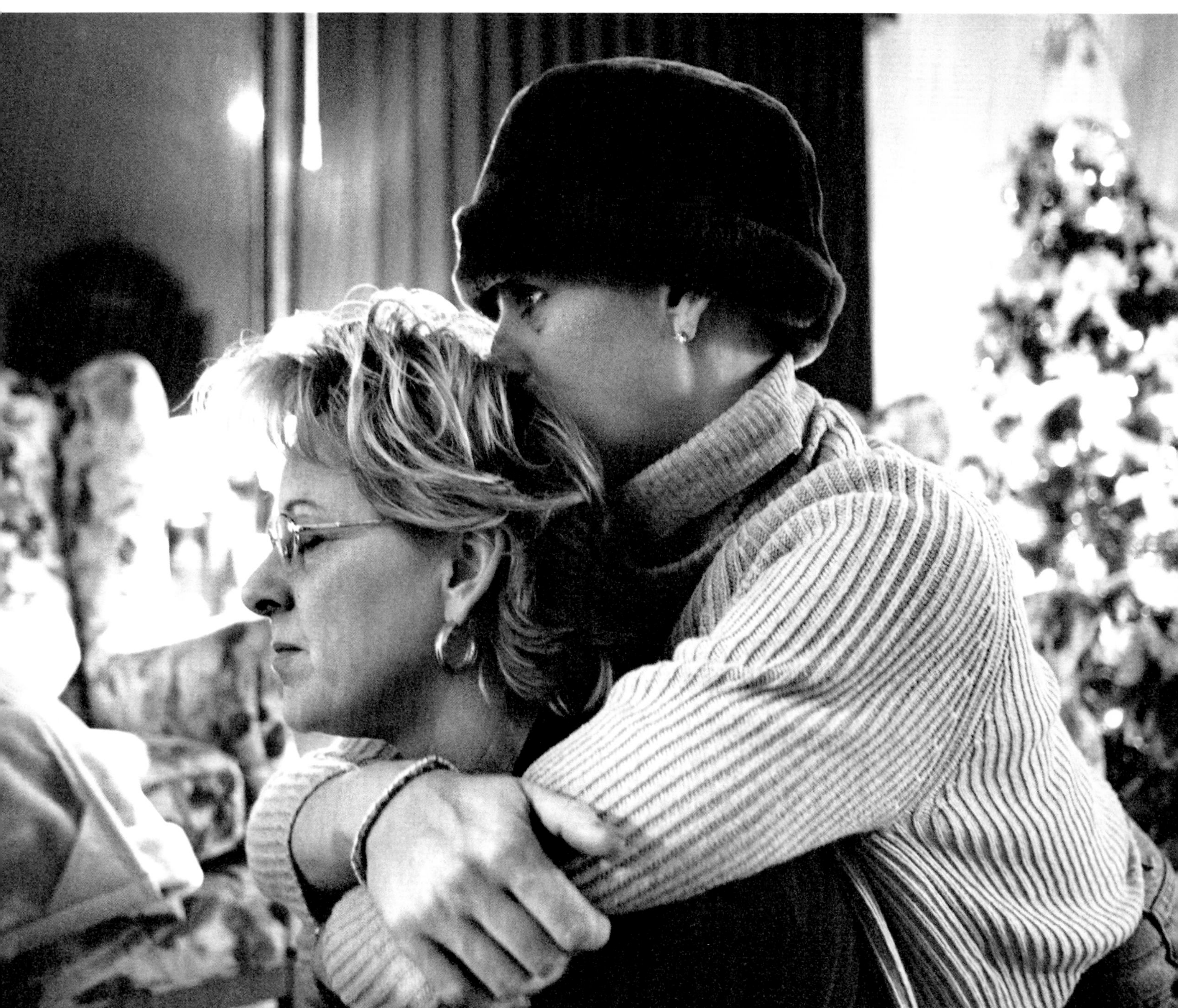

Barb and Tracy watch one of Barb's television ads.

Thursday, December 19. The *National Post* featured Barb on its front page. Barb's e-mail box filled up with notes from across the country.

"*Wow* is the only word that comes to mind on what you are doing during this time in your life," wrote Sheri Gauthier of Kingston, Ont. "When many would curl up in a ball and cry, you are helping others realize the dangers of smoking."

"To turn such personal pain to such a public issue deserves applause," wrote Jennifer Cairns-Burke of Charlottetown, PEI. "Listening to my mother's gravelly voice now, she who never lit a cigarette, but lived with my father for 37 years, is infuriating. He is a chain smoker, 2-4 packs per day, still. I also watched my mother-in-law, father-in-law, and two brothers-in-law die of lung cancer from smoking."

"Once I was done reading the article I took my cigarettes from my pocket and threw them in the garbage," wrote John Frayn of Edmonton. "I then cut the article out and will retain it for future reading when I am desperate for a cigarette (which will inevitably happen) and I need the same encouragement to quit."

"Barb is one person who might be able to reach my kids," wrote Kathryn Speck, an Edmonton school teacher. "She seems to have a God-given power to strike a chord with young kids."

Other big news organizations now wanted Barb. CBC Newsworld called to ask if she'd keep a weekly video diary. Her crusade was the topic on an open-line show in Winnipeg, where she was dubbed the Nicotine Nazi and a big hypocrite, because she was still smoking. On this day, though, she laughed off the criticism, encouraged as she was from all the e-mails. She had also received a call from New York, from a producer of *Good Morning America*, a show hosted by a prominent American journalist, Diane Sawyer, with seven million viewers. The producer wondered if Barb could appear on the show.

"I'm in shock," Barb told me in the morning.

Why did she think her crusade was getting so big?

"I can't explain it, other than I'm Irish and I got the gift of gab."

I hadn't planned to attend Barb's talk in Leduc, but her newfound celebrity and success created another hook for a news story. When I pulled up to the school, I saw a satellite truck parked in the lot, the Canadian Broadcasting Corporation ready to beam a hit on Barb's talk out on its national shows.

I sat for a moment in my parked car in wonderment.

Why *was* Barb so popular?

Part of it was her gift, as she said. She was loud and outgoing, but also distinctly feminine, full of charming, coquettish gestures — the tilt of her head, the batting of her eyelashes, the sweet smile, her hand on an arm, or touching a face. She called every man she met her 'budsie' and every woman 'babes' or 'sweetie.' Her hero was Princess Diana, Tracy pointed out to me, and like her idol, Barb had a way with strangers and with crowds. "Barb found the secret of how to make people love her."

But Barb's success was also related to her uniqueness, to her being a trailblazer.

Again, I wondered, why hadn't anyone else done this kind of work?

Maybe other dying smokers had tried to speak out,

but the time wasn't yet right, people weren't ready to listen. Or maybe no one had ever even tried. There'd always been a powerful taboo around cancer. I remembered my old boss, a smoker, a newspaper columnist, quite a crude man at times, but when it came to cancer, the 'c-word,' as he called it, he was cautious and respectful. It was a big deal when he wrote that a local big-wig had the disease.

Things changed, though, in the 1990s, with talk shows like *Oprah*, where people laid bare the details of their private lives. So much was coming out now that had once been kept secret, and North America was also becoming increasingly anti-smoking, and ready to enact tough anti-smoking laws.

It had all come together in Barb's crusade: a woman ready to talk, a world ready to listen.

"You know what I eat? Water!" Barb shouted out at Leduc's Christ the King school.

She was angry, raging. "If you think this is a farce, *think again*! Every day I wonder if my aorta is going to blow or if my brain is going to blow. That's the reality."

Afterwards, Barb was again mobbed by girls. The high school boys hung back, watching intently, trying to control their emotions. The rawness of Barb's talk had clearly moved them.

One boy, 15-year-old Luc Caouette, stood with his older brother Marcel. Luc was one of the school's tough, cool kids. He had sideburns, a goatee, spiked hair. He'd been smoking since he was nine, he told me, and was up to a pack a day.

"I thought smoking was cool, just like everyone else."

But now he had a bad cough, he said, and sometimes trouble even breathing.

"Everyday it gets worse, man, the breathing, the coughing. One day, I would be just like Barb and I don't want to do that."

What did he think of Barb's message?

"I think she's doing the smartest thing anybody could do. It touched me, man. Screw smoking, man. I'm going to carry on with my life."

Luc pulled a pack of cigarettes from his pocket and crumpled them up. He wasn't a shy kid, but he seemed proud, not the type to make a show of his emotions around Barb. I knew she would want to talk to him, though, so I told Luc he should show Barb what he'd done. At once, he approached her. He said nothing, but his eyes glistened. He handed her the crumpled pack. His face and body were rigid as he tried to suppress tears.

Just then, Barb teared up herself, something I'd never seen her do before with the kids.

"Oh, I'm so proud of you," she said, then hugged Luc close. "I told you the world has phenomenal opportunities, and now you're going to make it happen."

With that, she started to cry openly. "I don't want you to die the way I'm dying. You know what? You're going to make it. This is the best present," she held up the crumpled package. "You just made my Christmas."

Monday, December 23. With all the talk that Barb might not make it to Christmas, Mackenzie was downcast as the holiday approached. She expected her mother to die at any moment. It didn't help anyone's mood at the Tarbox household that today was the anniversary of Michael's death.

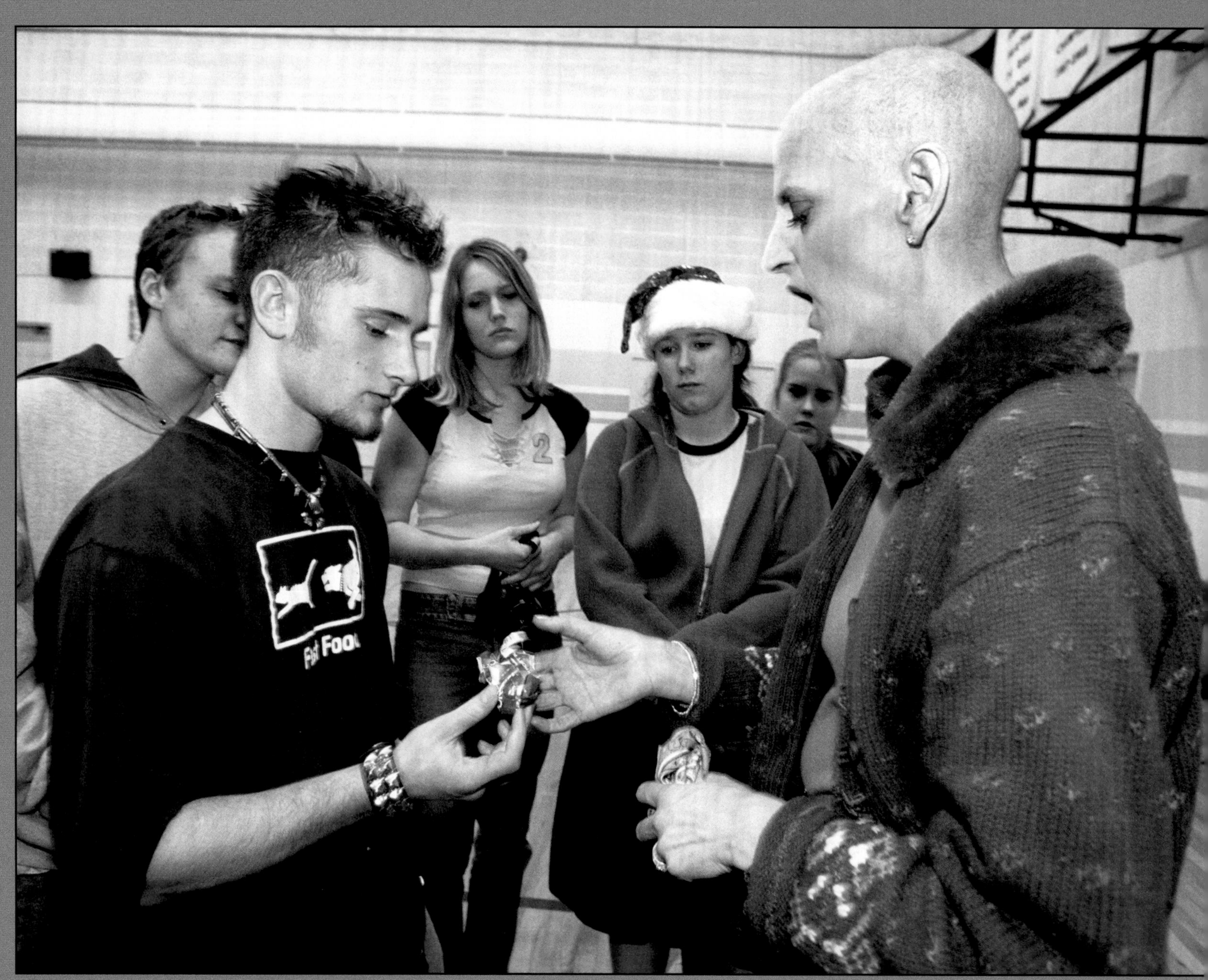

Luc Caouette hands Barb his crumpled cigarettes after hearing her speak at his school in Leduc.

Luc handed her the crumpled pack. His face and body were rigid as he tried to suppress tears.

Just then, Barb teared up herself, something I'd never seen her do before with the kids.

"Oh, I'm so proud of you," she said, then hugged Luc close.

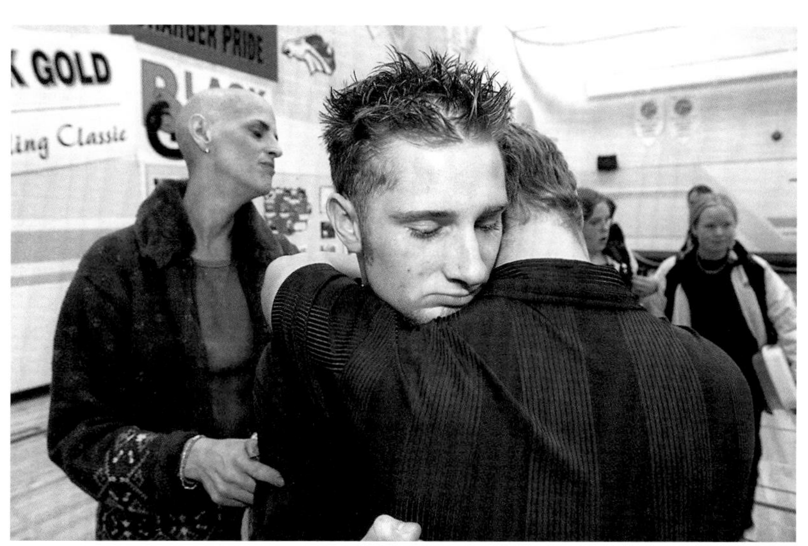

"I told you the world has phenomenal opportunities, and now you're going to make it happen."

Luc Caouette gets a hug from his older brother Marcel.

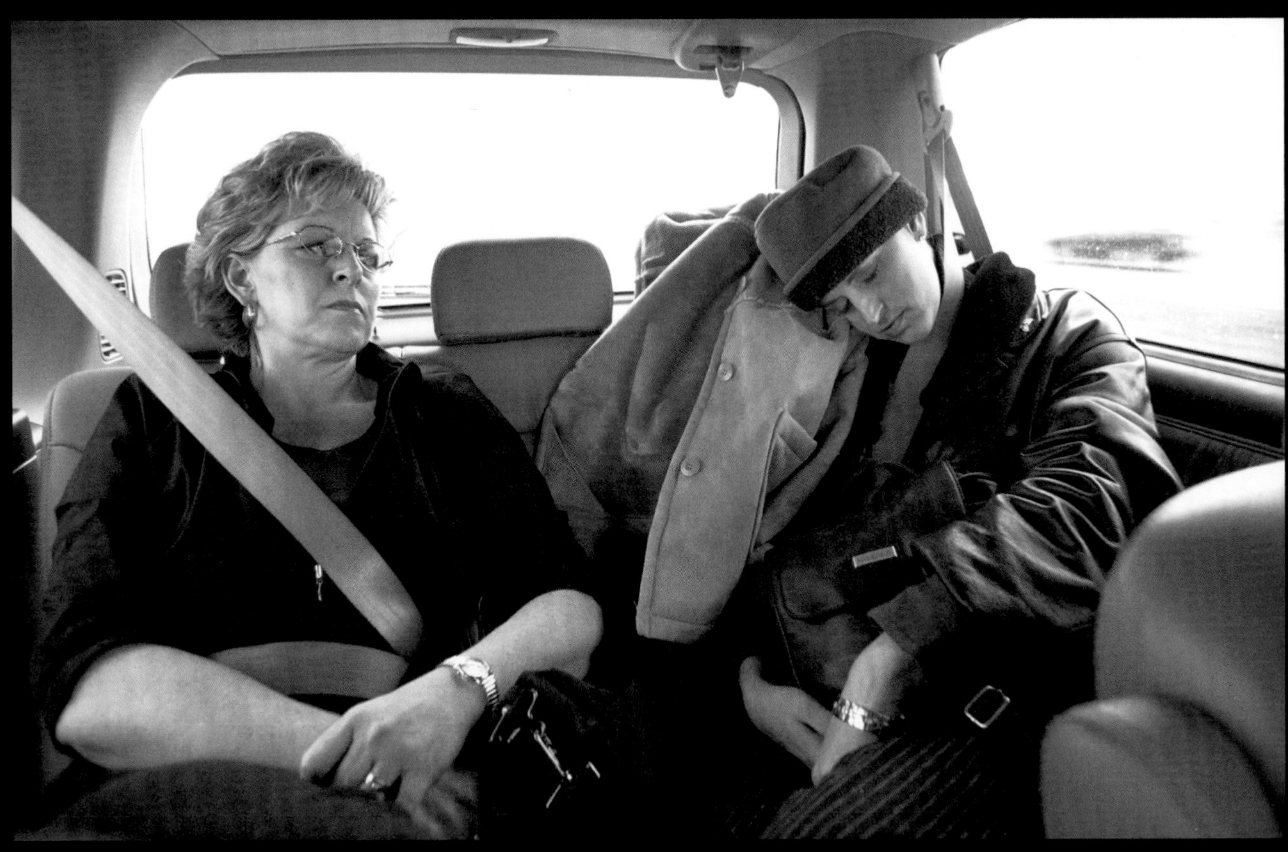

Tracy and Barb on their way back to Edmonton from a talk.

The Christmas season was always bittersweet, Barb told me, with so many sad anniversaries, Michael's death, then Patrick's. The family made sure to light candles for the two boys. "I've raised Mackenzie to think they're always with us," Barb said. "Always."

Tuesday, December 24. "Six weeks ago, I didn't think this day would come," radio host Al Stafford of CHED said on his Christmas Eve editorial. "On Remembrance Day, I met Barb Tarbox for the first time. . . Her doctors didn't think she would live until Christmas. She made it, and it looks like she's going to defy the odds and the experts for a while longer. . . The gift I will remember the most this Christmas is that my friend got one more Christmas with her family. And every day Barb Tarbox gets after that is one more gift she

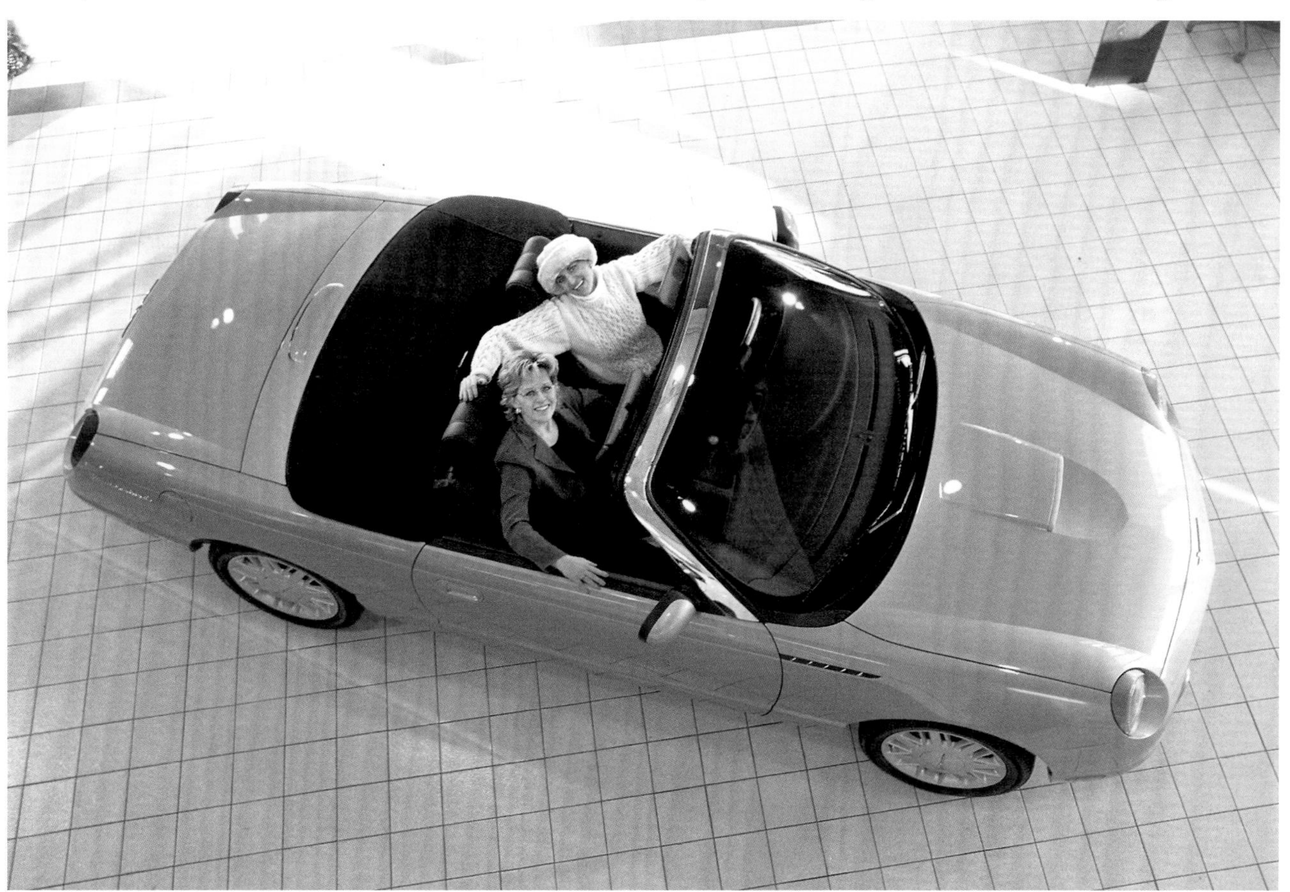

Barb and Tracy get together at Team Ford on Christmas Eve. Tracy's bosses at the car dealership gave Tracy unlimited time off to work with Barb and her crusade.

will use in ways most of us could never imagine."

Barb was driving when she heard Stafford talk. She had to pull over, because she'd burst into tears.

Christmas Day, Wednesday, December 25. Early Christmas morning, Barb was unable to sleep. The CBC had set up a camera in her living room for her video diary. She turned it on and started to vent. She'd made it to Christmas, made her goal, but that didn't make things better. She was still dying a stupid death.

Having vented, she felt on the verge of hysterical tears, knowing that this was certainly her last Christmas. Tracy was coming over for dinner, and Barb told herself, "I can't let Tracy watch me cry, because she'll burst into tears."

At dinner, Barb was able to eat some turkey, mashed potatoes, stuffing and gravy, but she got a painful heartburn.

Friday, December 27. Mackenzie was angry, argumentative, not doing things she was asked to do.

"That's OK," Barb said to me. "That's part of it. I don't like it. I hate it. But she needs more Mom attention. She has to accept this is happening."

Saturday, December 28. Tracy, Barb and I met for breakfast at the Delta Hotel with Graydon McCrea, an executive producer for the National Film Board, the federal government's film agency. McCrea had contacted Barb about making a film about her crusade.

The situation with Mackenzie had resolved itself, Barb told us as we waited for McCrea. She had broken down in front of Barb and wept. "I just wish you had never started smoking," Mackenzie had said.

Barb remembered how her own mother had been supportive when Barb was angry about her dying. Barb tried to do the same now. She and Mackenzie made plans for the future, how her favourite aunt would pick her up for school, take care of her, and she she would spend a lot of time with her cousins, Ashley and Nicole.

To take her cancer out of the picture, Barb also decided the video camera in the living room was too much, so she was going to ask CBC to take it away.

McCrea showed up. He was a rumpled, thoughtful man in his 50s, with a quiet sense of humour. Barb adored him at once. He said the NFB was looking for an anti-smoking story that would hit young girls. "It's the one area of the population where smoking continues to increase."

"That's great," Barb said. "If you can reach one child, we'd be forever grateful."

"Really, *you'd* be the one reaching them. We'd just be the mechanism."

Barb told McCrea she was best with grades seven to twelve. "I go in very aggressive and powerful. Every single school where I've been, I have left with hundreds and hundreds of hugs. There is not a school where you won't see tears, and you'll see the tears flooding."

Her goal had been to speak to 1,000 kids, she said, then 5,000, then 10,000. Now it was 20,000. "I just keep adding."

Opposite page: Barb opens her last Christmas present while Mackenzie holds onto an angel that Barb had given to her. This was their last Christmas together.

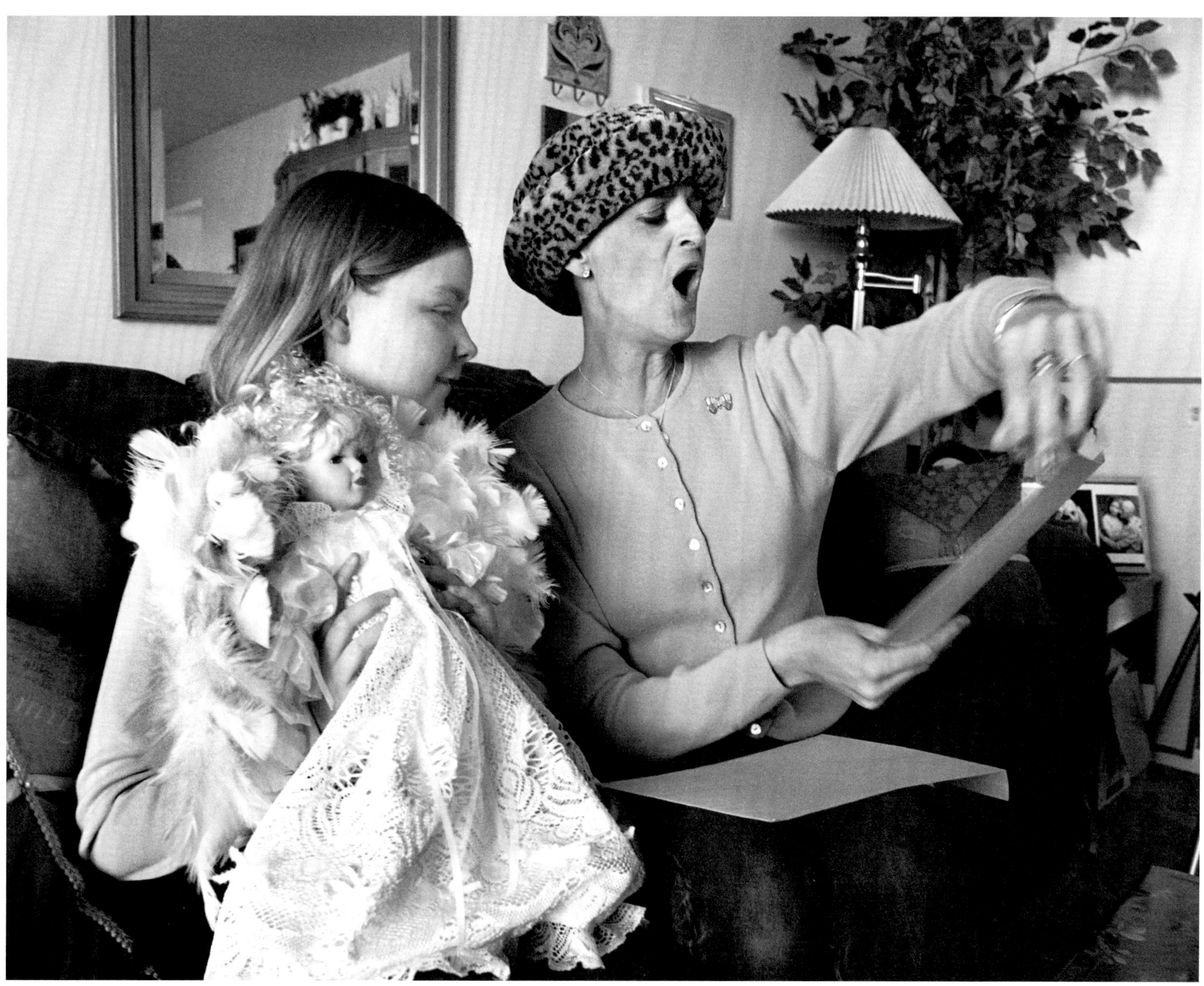

Barb turned to Tracy, then looked back at McCrea. "Without Tracy, this path, I could not have walked it," she said. "God has chosen this path for me, but he also sends his strongest angels to walk right beside you, and that's what he has done."

Tears formed in Tracy's eyes.

Barb next told McCrea about her meeting with the Caouette brothers, Luc and Marcel, in Leduc, and how Luc had passed her his crumpled cigarettes.

"I feel like I was touched by God Himself. What this young boy did to me, it was so touching."

Seeing the two teenagers had made her think of her owns sons, Michael and Patrick, and what they might have looked like if they had lived. "He had Michael's eyes," she said of Luc. "That was a gift from God, without a doubt. They were definitely sent from heaven for me, that's the way I look at it."

"Or maybe," McCrea said, "you were sent to them."

Monday, December 30. Barb e-mailed Greg, Tracy and me in the afternoon to say she wanted to book more schools in January. "I have given this a lot of thought, and although I know I was supposed to cut down on the schools I was visiting, which I did when I gave up that one day a week, I've decided to take it back. I look at it this way . . . I'll have plenty of time to RELAX. Now is not the time."

It struck me how Barb wrote to the three of us now as if we were a team. Even if I still felt somewhat removed, I was glad she felt that way. It felt good to be getting closer, to be a tight unit, the four of us, heading out on this crusade: Tracy taking care of details, me scribbling notes, Greg taking pictures, and Barb the star of the show, the tragic, irrepressible, delightful, driven star.

New Year's Eve, Tuesday, December 31. Barb visited Calder Bateman's downtown office to shoot film that would later be cut into a series of public service announcements. Greg accompanied her to take pictures. Craig Marler and Frank Calder looked on as Barb spoke, giving her little direction, save to tell her to speak on various topics, such as saying good-bye to Mackenzie, or the reasons she had started to smoke. Barb talked at length, with great passion, weeping at times, her words making a terrific impression on everyone in the room. As soon as the scene was over, though, she contained her emotions. "So how was that?" she asked matter-of-factly. "How did I do?"

It was as if she had flipped a switch, Greg thought. She could go from emoting to judging her performance in one second.

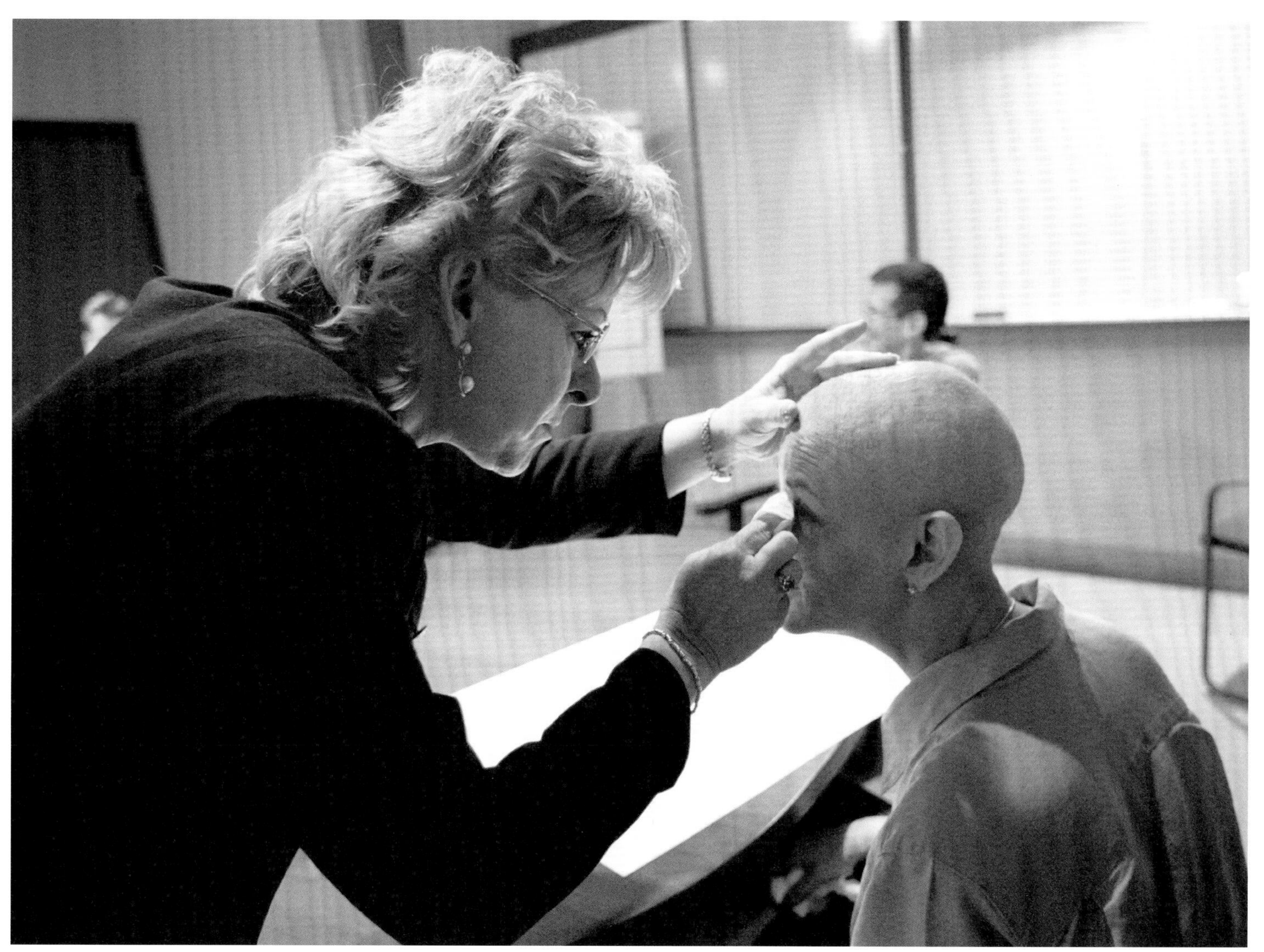

Tracy helps Barb with makeup while getting ready to film a series of public service announcement.

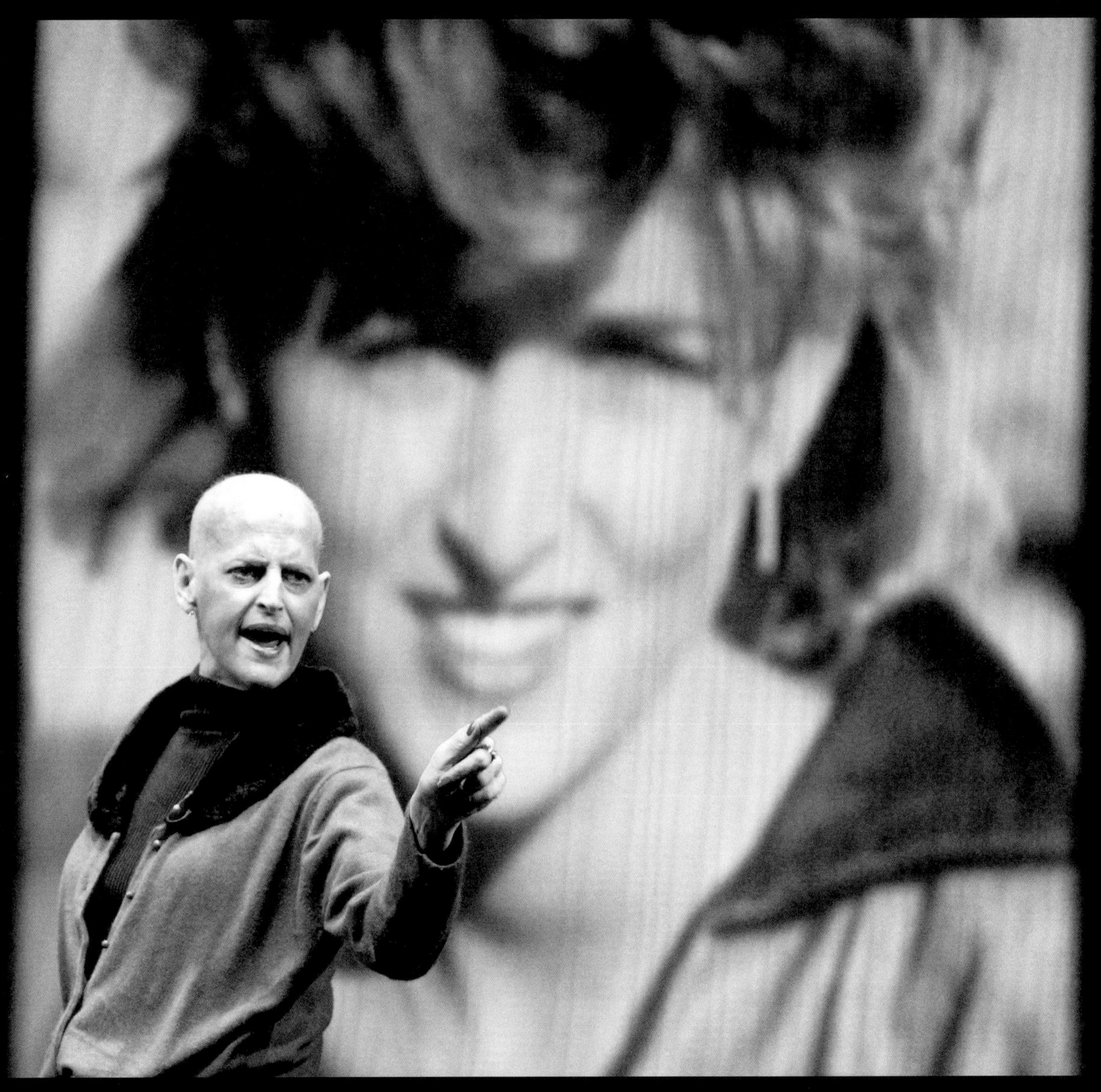

Barb speaks to over 1,000 kids at the Jubilee Auditorium while standing in front of a projected picture of herself taken shortly after she was diagnosed with lung cancer in September.

January

2003

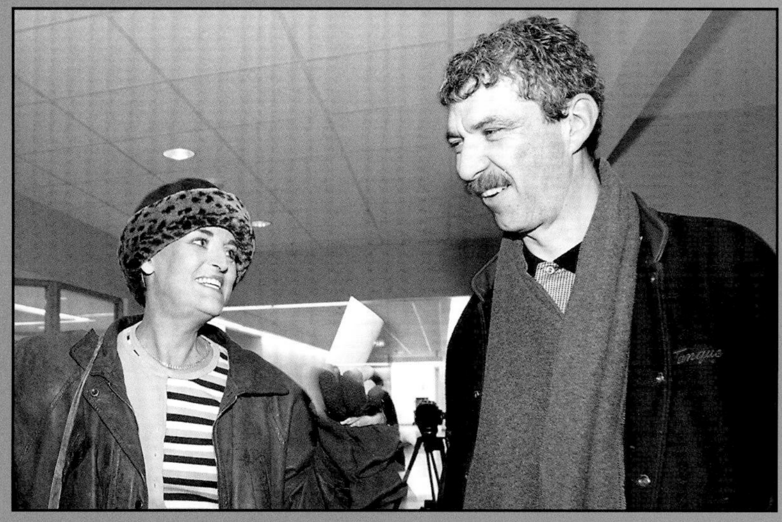

There is a stone there,
That whoever kisses,
Oh, he never misses
To grow eloquent.
'Tis he may clamber
To a lady's chamber,
Or become a member
Of Parliament.

Francis Sylvester Mahony

Tuesday, January 7. Through the holidays and early into the New Year, Barb pushed Tracy to book more schools and complained if things weren't set up exactly to her liking. At last, Tracy snapped back.

"I am not your fucking slave," she told Barb.

Barb wept and apologized. She realized she wasn't herself, she told Tracy. She was so tired now. It was hard to keep her eyes open, let alone get anything done. She was putting a lot of pressure on herself to keep going, but it wasn't working.

Wednesday, January 8. Almost every day, Barb got letters from admirers and from newly-converted ex-smokers. I asked to see them, so she started to forward them to me.

"I have been praying for you every day, knowing God is with you and is guiding you," read one from Earla Diletzoy of Edmonton. "He has given you a job and you are fulfilling it with grace."

Barb awoke with terrible pain in her ribs, coughing up mucous. She had a presentation planned for the morning, but she called up Tracy to have it cancelled.

Barb had no appetite now. When she walked through the mall, she would see people eating and she envied them. She remembered what it was like to be hungry, but that was all.

She was taking four morphine pills a day. She fell asleep in the bath. Her eyes looked droopy, tired. She shuffled like an old lady. Blood vessels on her legs looked like road maps. The surest sign of her distress was that she said she would have to cut back to two schools per week.

"There's so much weakness," she told Tracy. "It's overwhelming."

She talked about getting a blood transfusion as a pick-me-up.

"She looks awful," Tracy told me over the phone. "She looks dead. It's not how I want to remember Barb at all."

I talked to Barb in the evening. She seemed as positive as ever, and joked about how she hoped to look in heaven. She wanted to keep all her height, she said, but didn't want the same chest. "I'm going to be a wee bit greedy this time," she said and laughed. "Jaclyn Smith," she continued, referring to the curvy star from the old *Charlie's Angels* TV show. "She's classic, she's classic. But just the chest, that's all. I'm going to request that. But you watch, I'm going to be 4-feet, 8-inches."

Just then, I decided to confront Barb about her smoking during her pregnancy. At once, she admitted her lie, saying she had cut down, but hadn't stopped. Her sisters-in-law all smoked when they were pregnant, and they had no trouble, she said, though her mother, a smoker, had had a number of miscarriages. Barb had been on bed-rest during her own pregnancies to prevent the same. "It was simple to go down to five cigarettes when you're flat on your back," she said.

When I asked if her smoking might have led to her boys being born premature and sick, she went silent for a moment, then said she didn't think so, that miscarriages and pregnancy problems ran in her family.

I didn't think to say it right then, but smoking, too, ran in Barb's family.

Thursday, January 9. "My mother has smoked for 26 years," wrote 26-year-old Benjamin Georgy of

Edmonton to Barb. "I've begged her to quit, probably since the day I could talk. Just because of the wonderful things you've been doing for so many other people, my mom has finally decided to quit smoking nasty cigarettes."

In the morning, Barb's cohort — Greg, Tracy and me — all crammed into Dr. Fonteyne's small examination room, Barb up on the bed, me seated, taking notes, Tracy and Greg in the corner, Greg with his huge lenses.

"Can you get a blood transfusion just to feel better?" Tracy asked.

"No," Fonteyne said.

Barb told Fonteyne that she had tried to sit down on the toilet, but her butt was so skinny, she fell right in.

"OK, that's where my life has gone," she said. "I'm in the toilet bowl."

We all laughed.

As we were leaving the office, we passed a drug store on the main floor.

"Do you want to go and get a cane?" Tracy asked.

"No!" Barb huffed.

"Hey, *you* brought it up yesterday."

"No, I'm not ready yet."

"I was going to ask them if you wanted a walker."

"*A walker!* I want to go into one of my talks on a skateboard! I'd like to go do some window shopping."

"You want to go look at canes?"

"I'm not looking at canes! I was thinking of a nice outfit."

It struck me just then that Barb was always making jokes about her infirmities. More than that, even when she described her symptoms to me, Fonteyne or anyone else, she never had a whining tone. Later, I asked Barb about her positive attitude. She said she never wanted to be a downer. She had no room for self-pity, she said, not with a lifetime of smoking behind her. "I've done this to my body. I've done this to myself. But you know what is worse? I'm doing it to Mackenzie. . . I look at a nine-year-old, she's already had to bury her brother, and now her mom. Is that fair to her? So that's why I don't feel sorry for myself."

Her determination to stop others from smoking had helped her get over her nerves for public speaking, she said, but she knew her zeal sometimes pushed her over the line. For instance, Barb said, she'd recently stopped a cigarette-smoking teenager on the street and had beseeched her: "Please, I'm dying of lung cancer. Please, quit smoking."

The girl's face had gone all white, Barb said.

"You're dying from lung cancer?"

"Because of the cigarette."

The girl had just looked at Barb and said, "I'll try."

Barb told me that she knew exactly what that meant: "Trying is bullshit. Trying won't work."

Monday, January 13. After her medication was adjusted, Barb's appetite was rekindled. She made a roast on the weekend. She was back doing presentations. The only thing that kept her from filling out her calendar was the prospect of the New York trip; she needed to keep things open. Problems had come up over Barb getting health insurance for the trip. In the meantime, she visited a few schools and did numerous interviews. The CBC *National* was preparing a documentary on her and was filming her around the city.

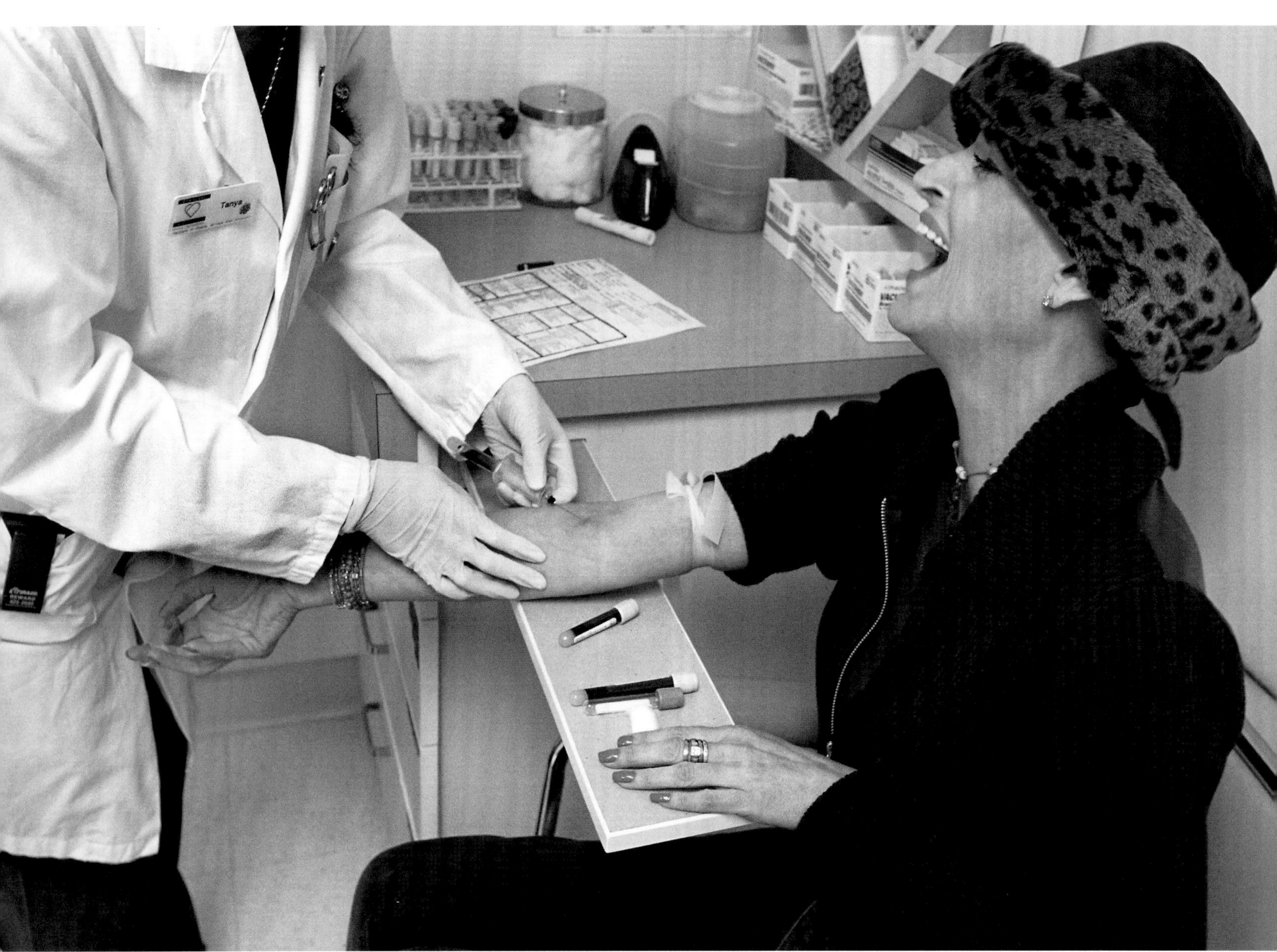

Barb laughs with her lab technician at the Grey Nuns hospital as she takes another blood test.

Listening to the CBC reporter interview Barb, Tracy was bothered by a new lie: Barb downplaying how much she was smoking. As the two headed out to interviews, Barb would chain-smoke in the car, but to reporters she claimed she was only having one or two a day.

Barb's lying made me reconsider one of things she liked to say, that she had the gift of gab. She certainly did, I now realized, but apparently she'd kissed the Blarney Stone a little too fervently.

Tuesday, January 14. The CBC filmed Barb speaking at Edmonton's Ottewell school. Pat came, standing near the exit, wanting to be unobtrusive. His eyes were riveted to Barb.

During the question-and-answer, a student asked if she smoked while she was pregnant.

"Yes, but I cut back," Barb said, much to my relief. "That's total honesty."

"How can you keep smiling knowing you're going to die?" a student asked.

"It's very, very difficult. I'm fortunate because I have my faith."

Afterwards, Pat told Barb that her speech was very good, but she had to watch Tracy more, because Tracy could give Barb signals that she was starting to repeat herself, as Barb sometimes did towards the end of her talks.

Wednesday, January 15. I could see that Barb and Tracy's views about religion and cosmology were deeply felt. Tracy offered to go through Barb's dream books with me, so we met for dinner at the Delta Inn.

Tracy told me the crusade and Barb's continuing deterioration were really hitting her hard. Tracy had been driving home from work and had started to weep. She had to stop by the side of the road to calm herself.

She pulled out the dream books. "Even if you think Barb is nuts, don't tell me that," she said. "She lives her life by her dreams. Her grandma did the same, her mom did, and now she does."

Barb jotted down the details of her dreams when she woke, believing God came to her in them, and if she could understand what they were saying, she would have clues about the future. The two of them would often sit up at Barb's house until 3 a.m. going through the books, and talking about Tracy's dreams, too.

In the last few years, there'd been many symbols of death in Barb's dreams, Tracy said. The dreams had been preparing her it, both she and Barb believed. In February 2000, for instance, Barb had had a spate of dreams where she was pale, a signal of mortality. On February 7 of that year, she dreamt about cameras, an airplane, a journey, luggage, baggage, running, cigarettes, a limo. In other dreams, she'd seen the Grey Nuns hospital, skeletons, corpses, cancer, chemotherapy, doctors, lungs, Tracy Mueller, x-rays, surgery, gravestones, chill winds, a fallen mirror. Many of these were signs of death, Tracy told me, but were also related to the current crusade.

When her own brother had died, Tracy had longed for him to come in a dream. Her sister had had one in which Tim showed up and said he was working with the RCMP to solve the murder.

"I wanted Tim to tell me who murdered him," Tracy said.

It never happened.

Barb dreamt of Tim, though. In the dream, she saw her twins, Michael and Patrick, playing under a tree. Barb got off a train, and wanted to run to the two boys, but in the dream Tim stopped her.

"It's not time yet," he said.

Thursday, January 16. "I am a lot like you, 39 years old, with two children that are my life and I have also smoked since I was 16 years old," Diane Morrison of Edmonton e-mailed Barb. "I have never tried to quit in my life and have only thought about it. You have touched me deeply. . . I have now picked a date to quit. I wish you and your family peace and comfort. You have made a difference. You are my hero."

With her health failing, Barb decided if she couldn't get out to see so many students, they could still be brought to her. The idea was to bring students from different schools together at a larger venue to hear her. The first two of these talks were set for today, in Fort McMurray, an oilpatch boomtown of 48,000 in northern Alberta. Barb was to talk to two large groups at two different schools, 2,000 students in total.

We flew over hundreds of miles of bush. I feared it would be blistering cold in Fort Mac, but the weather proved to be tolerable, about 15 below. We were met at the airport by two women, Kathy McKenna, chair of the Wood Buffalo Tobacco Reduction Coalition, and Melissa Ruryk, the group's co-ordinator. They told us Barb's message was desperately needed here. The city was Alberta's most addicted community. Thirty-nine per cent of adults smoked, compared to 25 per cent in the rest of Canada. Half of the city's children had tried a cigarette by the age of 12. Among teenagers, about 25 per cent were already hooked. At Fort MacKay, a nearby native community, many kids in the K-9 school started smoking in grade three.

"There's a lot of adult smokers here who influence the kids, lots of aboriginals, lots of blue collar, a lot of men," Ruryk said, as we headed into town. "There's also a major drug problem."

"It's the availability of money," McKenna said.

McKenna said she'd worried Barb would be too sick to make the trip. Barb told her she was just now feeling a lot better. She was able to eat more.

"It's frustrating, Barb," McKenna said.

"If you try to fight it, it becomes more of a battle," Barb said. "I'm not going to waste any energy on it. I knew it was coming, it's best just to accept it. I refuse to get hung up about it."

At our first stop, Father Patrick Mercredi high school, a teacher told me that smoking was rampant. Older teens, known as *breakers*, would buy up cigarette packs, then break them up, selling the smokes one by one for $1 to younger children, who were prohibited from purchasing the product at stores.

Barb was met at the door by many admirers, including town councillor Phil Meagher, the principal of Fort McMurray Composite High. "I think Barb is one of the bravest people I've ever met," Meagher told me. "My hero is Terry Fox and she ranks right up there with him."

It was quite the compliment. In the pantheon of Canadian heroes, Terry Fox was near the top. A statue of him had been erected in Ottawa. Fox had had cancer, a tumour in his leg. He had set off on a walk across Canada to raise funds for cancer research. He made it half-way before his health collapsed and he died.

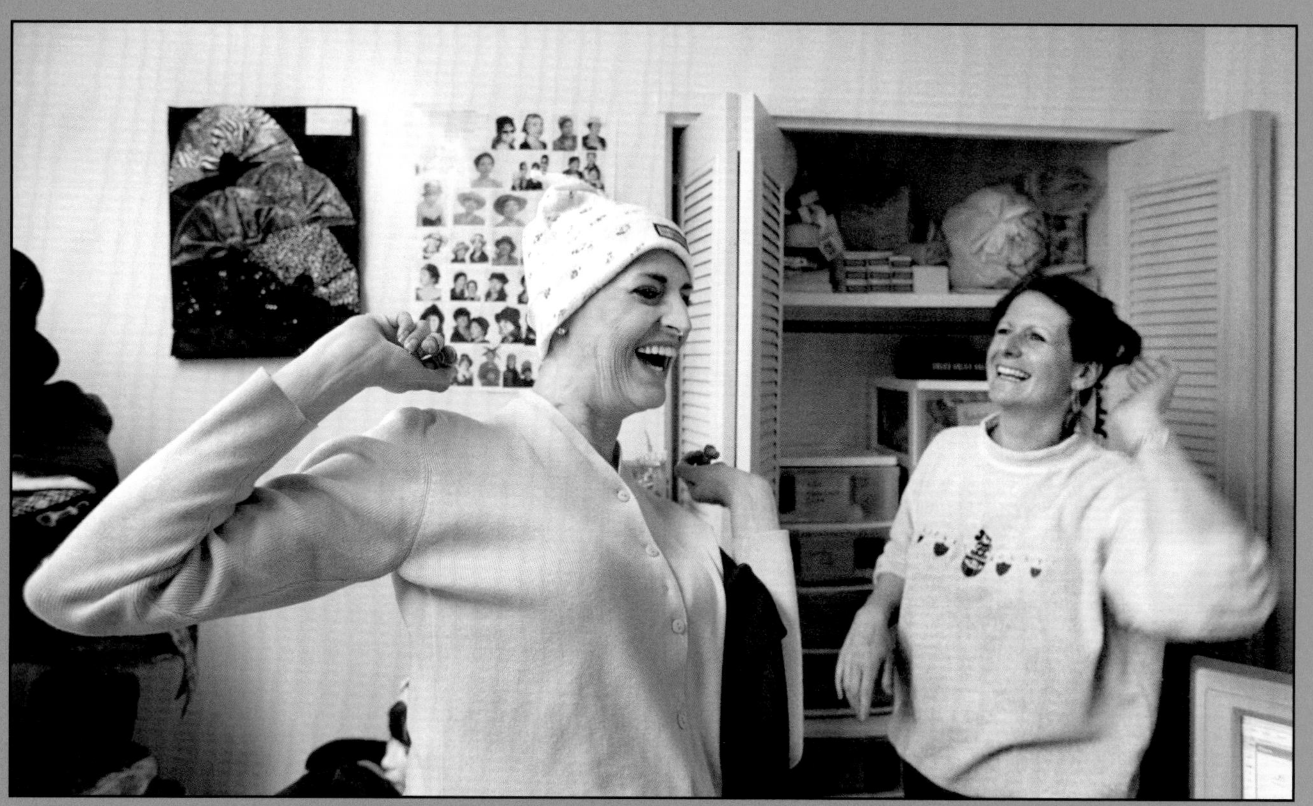

Barb tries on new hats made by Linda Finstad, a hat maker.
Barb loved hats and received a bag full of new ones from Linda.

Barb was introduced at Father Patrick Mercredi as a "blessed messenger from God." When she spoke this time, she had a cane in her hand. She told the kids about her weakness and her weight loss. "This outfit is my nine-year-old daughter's. I borrow her clothes now." Next, she spoke of her black and rotting flesh. "If you think there is anything on the market that can hide the smell, think again."

At our next stop, Westwood high school, I decided to change my usual pattern of sitting next to Tracy and instead took a seat in the stands, where the students were to sit. They filed in, chattering, looking about, changing seats, not thinking about Barb or her message. Instead, they were focused on what was really important to them at that moment: *Who will I sit beside? Where will I fit in?*

The teenage girls, wearing ties like pop star Avril Lavigne, talked and whispered and checked out the other girls, pretending not to see the boys. The boys, wearing tuques and sullen expressions like rapper Eminem, slouched in lumps, surrounded by their buddies, thinking this was all they needed in the world to be OK.

In front of the teens, sizing them up, Barb stood. To them, she appeared an oddity, a strange, stork-like woman with glittering eyes, wearing a hat indoors, wearing a bit too much make-up. Even as she got into her talk, most were still tuned out, whispering, fidgeting, much to my annoyance.

But then, Barb shifted gears, raising her voice: "I want to tell you guys that right here, right now, you guys are looking at *the world's biggest idiot*!"

That shut them up.

That always shut them up.

A moment later, Barb whipped off her hat, to reveal her baldness. The teens gasped. It was a startling, unforgettable image: shrunken body, sunken eyes, unfailing spirit.

Just then, I thought back to principal Meagher's comparison to Terry Fox. Even 20 years after his death, a strong image of Fox stuck in my head: a one-legged man struggling against the vastness of Canada. That image said it all: heroism, cancer, Canada. And now the image of Barb standing bald-headed before the students worked in a similar way: heroism, cancer, children.

Her talk reduced many of the kids to tears. Some of the girls held hands. One girl had her head down and was embraced by another. In the end, the two fled from the auditorium.

The students stood and cheered for Barb when she was done. The usual mob surrounded her afterwards. Instead of watching this scene, I tracked down a teacher and asked where the kids smoked at the school. I was directed out a side door. A few kids stood there in the cold, puffing away, including Nicole Stubbert, a 14-year-old who had been smoking for two years. Even as Barb was finishing her talk, Stubbert had been thinking of coming out here to light up. Barb had made her think about her habit, she said, but that's all. "I've tried to quit, but I just kept smoking."

"It scared the shit out of me," said another smoker Josh Evans, 17, who said he'd been at it for four years. "How she got cancer and all that."

This coming Friday, Evans said he was going on the patch. "Today is my last day."

In the evening, reporter Judy Piercy's documentary on Barb ran on the CBC *National*.

Friday, January 17. "Your talk was the only thing that has ever gotten through to me and made me want to quit smoking," student Danielle LeBlanc from Father Merc high school e-mailed Barb. "I bawled when I was there listening to you. . . I started (smoking) when I was nine and now I'm 14. That's almost six years and I'm still a kid. Like, I'm not proud of it at all because all of my little friends that I tried it with have quit. They are dancers and models. I'm just sitting here on the sidelines thinking, 'What the hell was going through my mind?'"

Sunday, January 19. E-mails flooded in as a result of the CBC documentary, including one from 44-year-old Joan Dundas of Brock University in St. Catharines, Ontario, who'd smoked for 20 years. "Friday's broadcast was emotionally wrenching and too close to home for me. While watching it, I decided that my daughter would help me shred my remaining cigarettes. . . My deepest thanks to Barb, a true angel."

Jason Bruckal of Vancouver, B.C.: "We are often unclear as to what it means to be Canadian, but Barb would be my definition. Her selfless drive to improve others' lives on a volunteer basis, and making the most of what she has, is an example to be followed."

And Bonnie Walline of Innisfail, Alberta: "I started smoking when I was 14 years old because of pressure from my boyfriend. I wanted so bad to fit in and be like the rest of the crowd. I'm 46 years old and I wish I had known then what I know now. I would never have started. Two weeks ago, I quit smoking again, and I'm determined for it to be for good this time. You've done this for me and I thank you."

Monday, January 20. The downtown Rotary Club of Edmonton set up Barb's biggest talk yet, busing in students from Edmonton's inner city schools, 1,200 in all, to the Jubilee Auditorium, an aging but elegant concert hall.

I met Barb in the performer's lounge. She was tickled that various star singers had prepared for their shows in this room over the years. She'd had a rough weekend, she said. At one point, she'd spent 20 minutes searching for her keys, then realized they were in her hand. On Sunday, she'd had her worst seizure yet. She felt dizzy, upside down. It felt as if the seizure came from outside, invading her through her left cheek. The smell seemed to go right to the middle of her body. It made her feel like she wasn't part of this world.

She was now back on high doses of anti-seizure medication. "I feel great today," she said.

The *Good Morning America* trip looked like it had fallen through, Barb said. Travel arrangements never could be finalized. She had given up on it so she could schedule other cities.

The NFB showed up to film her speech. Craig Marler of Calder Bateman had set up a slide show to go along with Barb's talk, huge images flashing up on a screen behind her as she talked, Barb with Mackenzie, Barb with Tracy, Barb in radiation therapy, Barb with a full head of hair.

Barb had shaped her message — with its focus on cancer causing not just death, but also ugliness and baldness — to tweak the vanity of teenaged girls. Canadians of all ages quit smoking at ever-increasing rates during the 1990s, except for teenage girls, who were starting to smoke more than ever before.

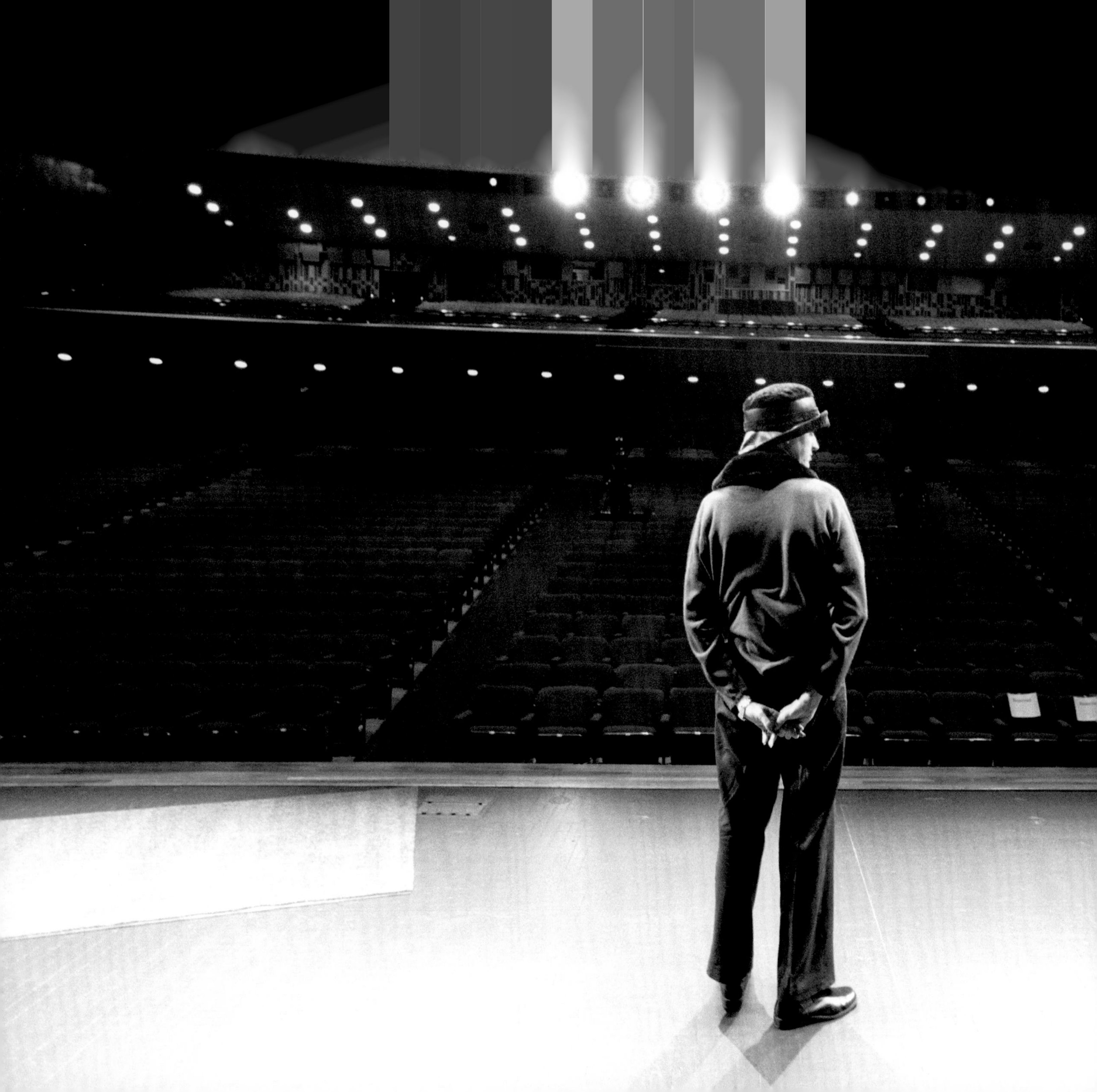

Barb takes a look around the Jubilee Auditorium before the inner-city kids arrive for a talk hosted by the downtown Rotary club.

Smoking-related cancers were becoming much more common in women. In 2001, lung cancer killed more women than breast cancer: 7,400 to 5,500.

After Barb's talk that day, a group of girls stood in the foyer, waiting for their bus. Jessica Schindel told me she badly wanted a cigarette. She'd been smoking since she was 12, she said. She was 15 now, and smoked half a pack a day. "I want to light a cigarette right now. But I'm not going to. I'm going to try to quit."

"No man," said her friend and smoking buddy Anna Moulden-Griffith. "We're not going to *try*. As of now, we are official non-smokers."

"It hurts for me to see Barb Tarbox like that," Schindel said. "I'm trying to make the change, but I don't know how to. The only thing stopping me is the weight issue, and that all my friends smoke around me. Being around other kids who are smoking, it makes me crave them. When I'm close to quitting smoking, a bunch of friends will come over and they'll all say, 'Here, have one,' and I'll say, 'OK.' I guess I kind of give in."

The girls exclaimed over the shots from the slide presentation of Barb with a full head of hair. It was all the more horrible for them when Barb suddenly revealed her bald head.

"I was like 'Oh my God!" Moulden-Griffith said. "It totally shocked me. I couldn't believe that smoking would do that. I couldn't deal with that."

What would she do if she lost her own hair to radiation treatments?

"I'd probably harass smoking companies until the day I die, just like Barb is doing."

Tuesday, January 21. The e-mails kept flooding, this time from students who'd been at the Jubilee. "I had a mom that smoked and died when I was five," wrote one of them, Avery Powder. "Just before she died, I wrote a note saying to get well soon. I was going to give it to her the next morning, but she passed away, so now I have two reasons not to smoke."

Tracy told me her co-workers at Team Ford were razzing her. Someone put an inflatable doll at her desk, since she wasn't using it much. It was all good natured, but Tracy was starting to fear that she might lose her job. The auditors were coming in at the end of January and the books had to be ready. At least her husband Werner was really coming through for her, Tracy said, picking up the kids from school, dropping them off, making supper.

Friday, January 24. The debate about Barb's worth as a crusader heated up on the letters page of the *Edmonton Journal* after one reader, Mike Powell, suggested she be awarded the Order of Canada: "Anyone who makes a massive attack on a disease that afflicts thousands of Canadians is a true hero in my estimation. Such a person is Barb Tarbox."

Not everyone agreed.

"The Order of Canada was designated for lifelong achievements; having smoked for 20-plus years does not qualify," wrote Rob Pinard of Edmonton.

And Vivian Stanley of Edson wrote, "Barb doesn't look or sound 'weak' or 'sick,' but she is getting all the sympathy and money she wants, braying about the evils of cigarettes. If she's that sick, wouldn't she rather be home with her husband and daughter? . . .

Or don't they care that you're never home?"

And another letter writer, Hannibal Wolf: "I see for Tarbox on the horizon a miraculous remission followed by a claim of divine intervention (isn't it always). Tarbox is entirely a media creation. . . Anyone stupid enough to believe her propaganda is just that: STUPID!"

Finally, Louise Sauter of Edmonton wrote to the CBC. "What I can't understand, why Barb is telling all these people to stop smoking, and I understand she is still SMOKING!"

Monday, January 27. To help out Tracy, Greg's ex-partner, Donna Gingera, an Edmonton public relations specialist, offered to start handling Barb's correspondence and scheduling. Donna pushed the crusade to a new level. First, she contacted the federal government, Health Canada, which agreed to start footing the bill for Barb and Tracy's travels. With that funding in place, Donna went to work scheduling events in Ontario, British Columbia and Quebec. She quickly booked $40,000 in flights.

Tuesday, January 28. Barb got a letter from an Ottewell student Jarrett Brown: "My grandma, dad, uncle and aunt quit smoking after I told them about you. My grandma and aunt gave in to the dreadful things and started to smoke again, but the rest are keeping strong. I've tried smoking and it tastes awful. I think that I will never start smoking."

A new issue had come up with Barb, the most troubling one yet for Tracy: money. Barb had said she never wanted to be paid for her talks, but now she was talking to both Tracy and Donna about asking for a fee, a dollar per student. The money wouldn't go into any special fund, Barb said, but to her, and she would direct it to various charities. Of course, there would be no way to verify that, and when Tracy and Donna suggested to a few schools that they should pay Barb in this manner, the administrators flatly refused.

But Barb continued to pester for the money. Tracy was appalled. She was doing all this for free, out of friendship for Barb. If Barb wanted money, that would change the whole equation.

"I'm not doing it," Tracy e-mailed me. "I said, 'No, *you* can say it. I'm not saying it. I'm not doing this for any money and you weren't doing it for money either.'"

Tracy wondered if the problem was that Barb needed money. She asked Barb, who admitted that was the case. Tracy lent her some.

Thursday, January 29. Two University of Calgary medical professors made an interesting proposal to Barb, suggesting that after her death, they make slides of her diseased body and tumours for education purposes.

"I'm doing it," Barb told me over lunch at a Whyte Avenue restaurant, Tasty Tom's. "What else could I do with my body? I could cremate it. And it will be cremated in a year's time. Some of the ashes will come back, and we'll mix it with Patrick and Michael and it will be buried."

For a year, though, her body would be studied inside and out, Barb said. "By God, they're bound to find something in this body, that's what I think."

"A big heart," Tracy said.

Earlier that morning, Barb had spoken at another junior high to 500 kids. She told us she was looking ahead to the next month and her numerous trips across Canada.

"It's insanity," she said.

"To put it mildly," said Tracy, less excitedly.

Barb ordered a cheeseburger and coke. The medication to increase her appetite was working.

Even though she ate, Barb was still losing weight, the tumours sucking all the energy out of her. Her legs had become so swollen she had to cut her jeans to get into them.

I asked Barb about some of the recent criticism, and whether she thought she was still effective as a spokesperson, even if she was smoking.

"If I had somebody come in when I was 13 and said what I am saying, I would have run from the cigarettes," she said. "I would have looked at her and said, 'Oh my God!'"

Most people were supporting her, she said. She would go to a mall and be surrounded by well-wishers and people who wanted a hug. "I absolutely love it. That gives me strength to keep going."

I next asked Barb about the money issue. It had all been a misunderstanding, she said. She didn't want any money for herself, but schools had been asking to make donations on her behalf, and she just wanted to make sure the money went to a charity of her choice.

"Did I become rich from developing lung cancer? No. It's not why I'm doing this."

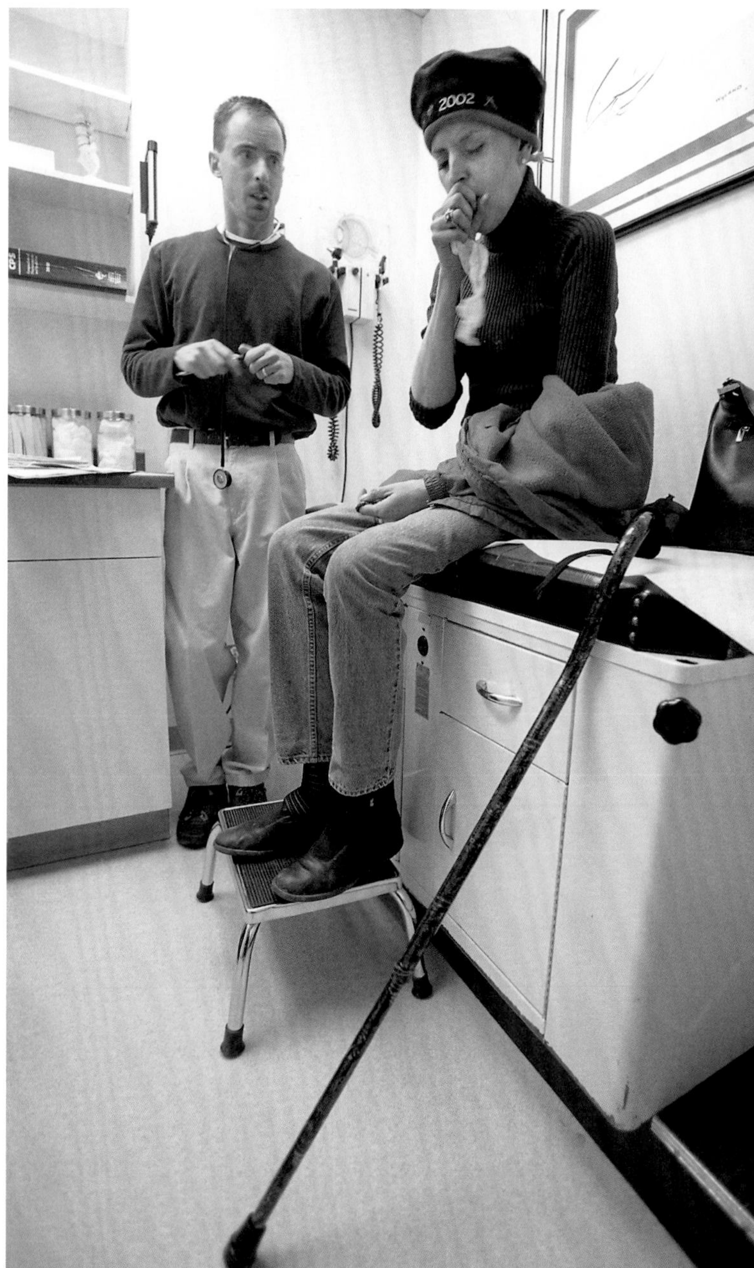

Barb liked to call Dr. Douglas Fonteyne "the most phenomenal doctor in all of Canada."

Friday, January 31. When Tracy looked at the travel schedule for February, she felt sick. Trips were planned to Red Deer, Toronto, Ottawa, Montreal, Grande Prairie and a number of smaller centres. At the same time, Tracy had to prepare for Team Ford's year-end audit.

"I hate it," she told me over the phone. "I'm in panic mode right now. I asked Barb for some of her morphine and she wouldn't give it to me."

Again, Tracy was upset at Pat for not doing more. "I can't say I'm enjoying it at all. We did our 27th presentation yesterday, and that's a lot. And that's not including the nine coming up here."

Tracy was now questioning why Barb wanted to be out speaking so much, instead of at home with Pat and Mackenzie. "I don't know if she's trying to run from something, but she wants to be somewhere every day."

It seemed reasonable to me that Barb would want to take her crusade as far as it could go, and I didn't think there was anything wrong or pathological about her relishing her newfound glory. Still, I sympathized with Tracy.

In the past month, I'd felt myself becoming wrapped up in Barb's crusade, too, not wanting to miss a talk, and not wanting to be away on weekends in case something happened with her health. I knew that my work should never come before my family life, and I was determined it wouldn't happen, but I could feel the unpleasant strain, the nagging call to do more with Barb.

Greg felt this strain even more strongly. He was having trouble sleeping, thinking about Barb and all he had to do, such as finally getting that photograph of her without any cosmetics on her face. His stomach was giving him pain. He feared he had an ulcer.

Of course, for Tracy the strain was worst of all. Barb was becoming irritable and demanding again, she told me. "She's not as compassionate about the time I need as she used to be. . . It's getting quite intense. Sometimes I see 'Tarbox' on my phone and I don't answer it. I just let them take a message. Sometimes it's 20 or 25 calls a day. I just got to get through this. I find Barb and I snapping at each other quite often. I can only keep my mouth shut so long. I told Barb, 'If I didn't tell you what I think and disagree with you, what kind of a friend would I be?' I told her I'm not a 'No sir, yes sir' kind of person."

Barb's smoking remained an issue. "I have to go in and buy her smokes every day," Tracy said. "She's too embarrassed to do it. She doesn't want everyone to see her buying cigarettes. I said, 'That's stupid, give me $50. I'll do it.'"

The most recent presentation had been awful, Tracy said. The gym filled up late, cutting into Barb's speaking time. Afterwards, Barb had blamed Tracy for booking the school.

"I think she's getting bitter now. I can hear it in her voice. I see it more than I did. She knows the end is coming quicker. As of this morning, she went to the doctor and she had lost 41 pounds and that drastic weight loss does stuff to your mind, not only your body."

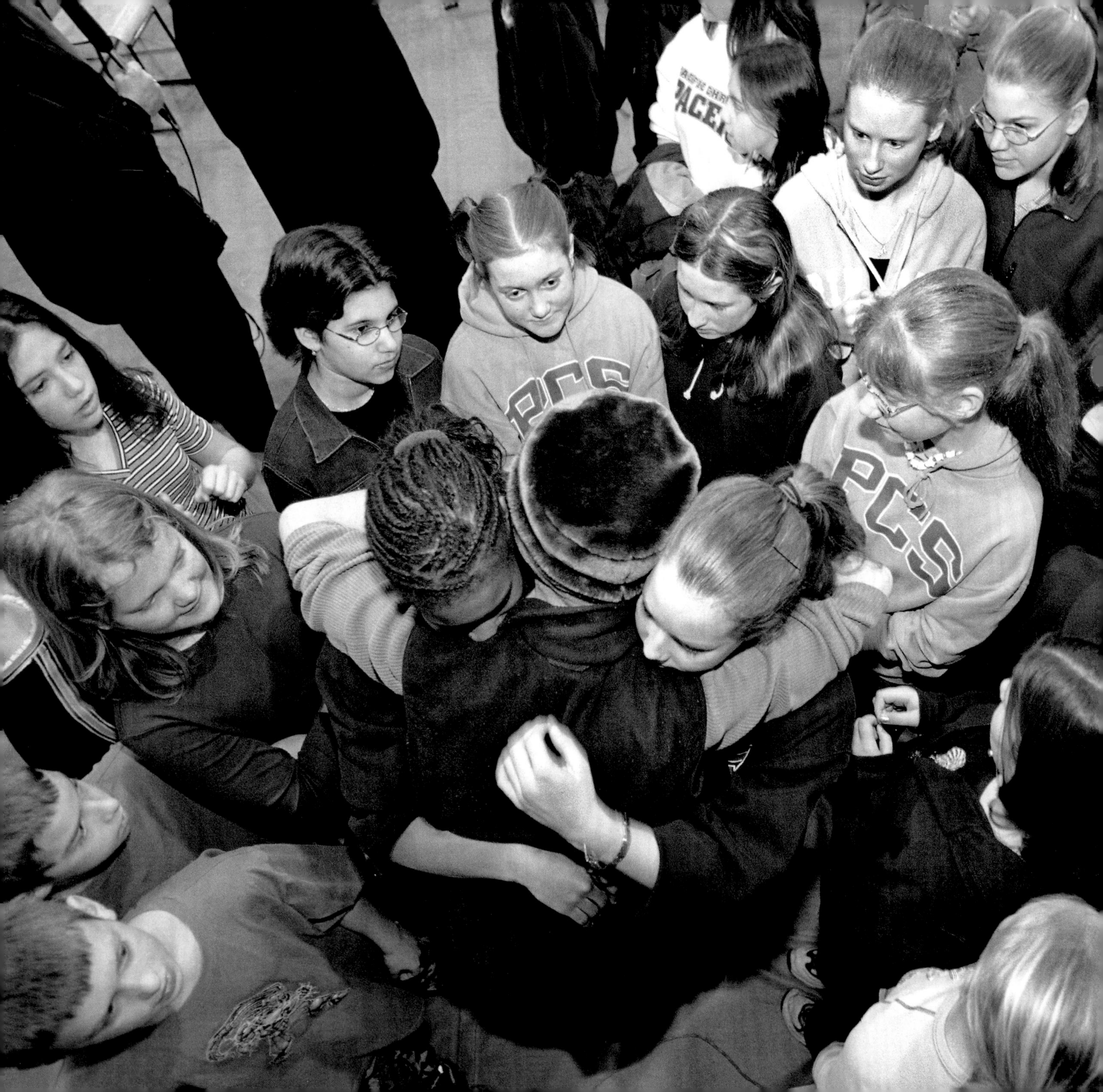
PCS
PCS

February

2003

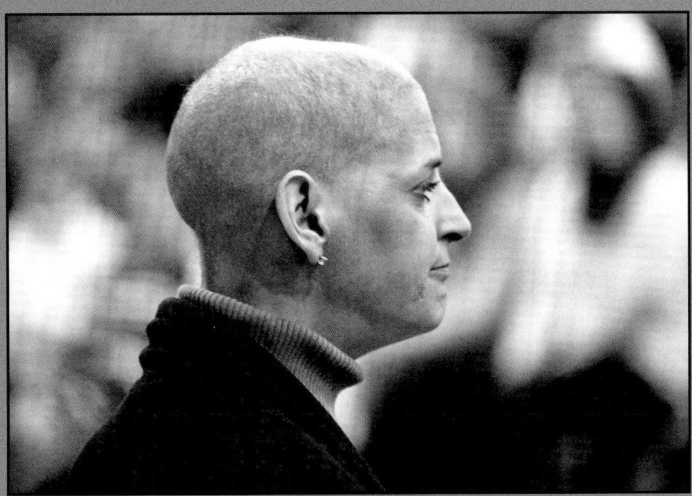

The saints differ from us in their exuberance, the excess of our human talents. Moderation is not their secret. It is in the wildness of their dreams, the desperate vitality of their ambitions, that they stand apart from ordinary people of good will.

Phyllis McGinley

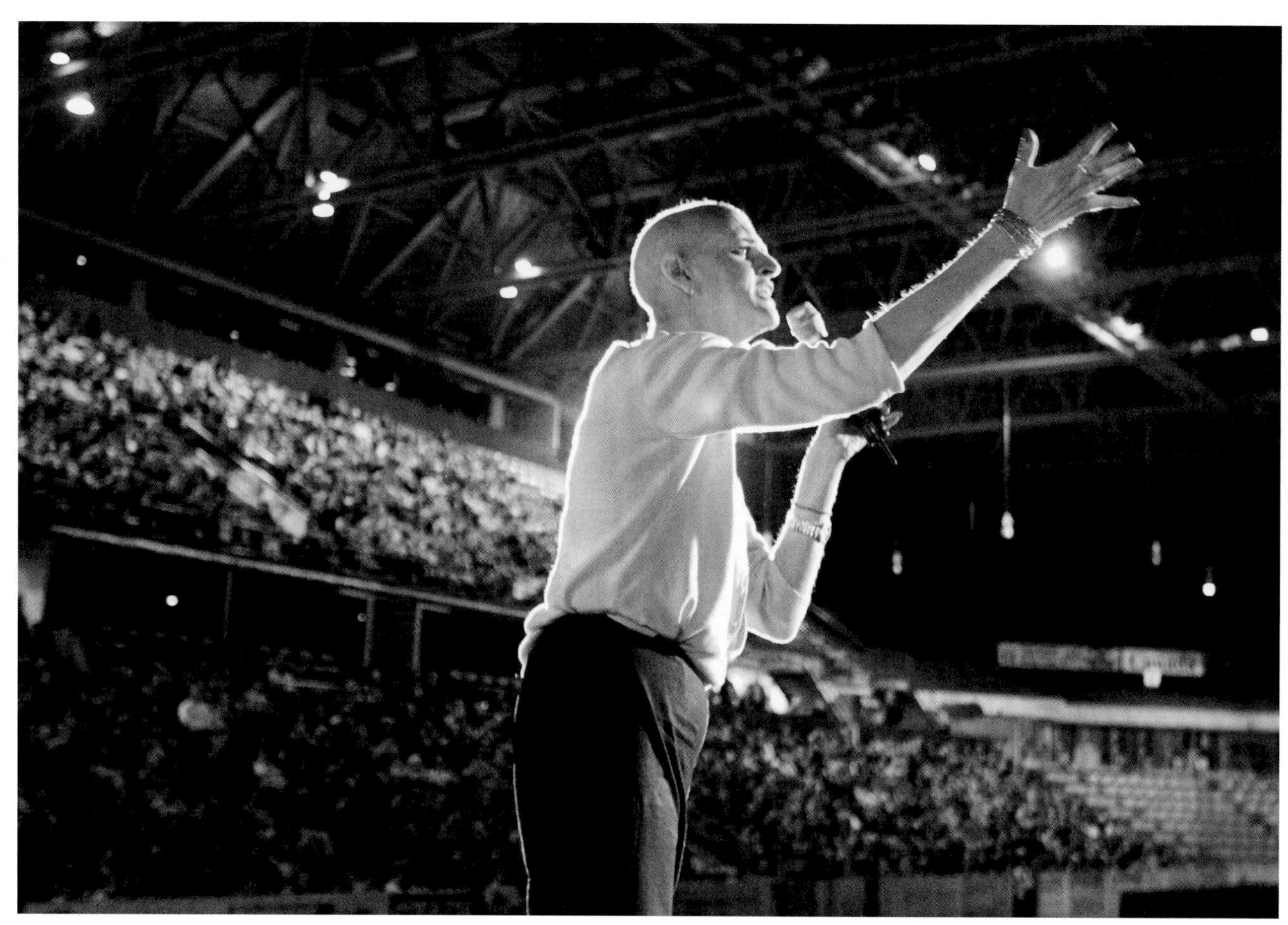

Barb talks to 4,000 people at the Red Deer Centrium arena.

Monday, February 3. I'd seen enough of Barb's presentation, and had other deadlines to meet, so I didn't go see her speak at Vimy Academy in Edmonton. She e-mailed me later, telling me she'd missed her 'wee brothers', the nickname she'd given to Greg and me. "I want to start seeing you at these presentations. It's not the same without you and Greg."

Wednesday, February 5. Teachers, parents and students all pressured Barb to do presentations. For example, a girl named Katie Thaller e-mailed to plead with Barb to present at her school, Riverbend junior high. "There are so many kids that smoke there. I am ashamed to admit that I am one of them. I shouldn't because my grandpa died of lung cancer. I hate the fact that I do. I hate going to school every day and at lunch seeing my friends and Grade Eights and Grade Sevens smoking too! Every time your story comes out in the news, my whole body goes numb and I feel like I'm going to cry. Will you please, please consider coming to my school."

And Breanne Fisher, a 13-year-old from Ottewell school, asked Barb to come to her house to convince her dad to quit smoking. She'd tried many times, Breanne said, including once when she called up a radio program to speak to Santa. "After asking for a new toy and a pair of shoes for my mom, I hesitated when Santa asked what I wanted for my father. Then when it came to me, it seemed like the best present of all. 'Could you please stop him from smoking?' That was almost five years ago and no real change has occurred. I think that he just doesn't feel compelled enough to do so, which really pains me."

Barb's talk today was to be for 4,000 students, all packed into the Centrium, the biggest hockey rink in Red Deer, a city 200 km south of Edmonton.

"Try to imagine that number: 4,000," Barb said. "I've got so many people to touch. We started out with 30 kids. Now it's 4,000."

Barb, Tracy, Greg and I sat down for breakfast at a Red Deer restaurant. We had driven around for some time before we found a place that allowed smoking. Barb ordered a coffee, along with bacon and eggs. She dumped ten packets of sugar into her coffee.

"She could be a blimpo," Tracy said.

"This is true," Barb said. "I try to have five or six Pepsis a day."

There was talk of a movie on her crusade, Barb told us. A Vancouver writer, Robert French, had contacted her. Barb was in a good mood, so Greg and I decided to press her about allowing Greg to photograph her with no make-up on.

I asked why she was procrastinating.

"I've loved make-up for 31 years," she said. "It's vanity."

But she'd still do it, she promised. The elevated veins had now spread from her legs to her stomach. "People never, ever talk about this. It's so gross and so hideous."

Barb excused herself to go the washroom. While she was gone, Tracy said the two of them had just had a big fight on the drive to Red Deer. Barb had promised to limit her presentations to two a week, Tracy said, but now was booked for four or five a week through February. She had even wanted to book a presentation on February 17, Mackenzie's birthday. Barb said they could just celebrate the following day.

It was all too much, Tracy said, and at last she had let Barb know how frustrated and tired she was. It was good to get her feelings out into the open.

"It took so much pressure off," she said of their fight. "I almost hated her. I thought, 'I can't stand being around you. I can't stand doing this. It's eating my life up.' "

I asked Tracy why she thought Barb was becoming so obsessed with her crusade.

It was a huge ego boost for Barb, Tracy replied. Barb was addicted to the attention. "Of course, she had zero attention before this. She was a stay-at-home mom, and she went from school to volunteering, then back home again. Now she's doing this and she's thriving on this. She absolutely loves it."

Tracy had told Barb to book nothing for March, that she'd had enough. "I said, 'You're obsessed. And I can't deal with it anymore.'"

Barb had agreed.

"I feel 100 per cent better," Tracy said. "I'm excited to go to Ottawa."

Students packed the arena. All of the grade six to nine public school children in Red Deer had been bused in for the talk. The event had the feel of a big game, or concert, or religious revival. Stage lights lit up Barb as she spoke, her every move and gesture projected onto a massive screen behind her. Her voice reverberated through the rink and, even in the last rows, children were moved to tears.

Immediately afterwards, Tracy and Barb jetted off to Ottawa, seemingly united once again.

Thursday, February 6. Health Canada gave Barb, Tracy and Calder Bateman's Craig Marler the V.I.P. treatment in Ottawa. They were put up in the posh Chateau Laurier and shepherded around by government officials. Health Minister Anne McLellan introduced Barb for her talk at Hillcrest high school

"Smoking affects many, many people," Barb told the crowd. "My mother died nineteen years ago when I was very young because she was a smoker for forty years. Let me personally tell you, there has not been a day in 19 years when I haven't thought of my mother. My father died 15 years ago. There hasn't been a day when I haven't thought of my father. And both my twin sons, incredible human beings, have both died. You better believe that smoking affects you."

Next stop was the House of Commons, where Barb lunched with McLellan, then went to the Prime Minister's Office and met briefly with Jean Chrétien. McLellan gave Tracy a hug for all the good work she was doing.

After lunch, Barb was introduced to the House of Commons. "I rise in the House today to pay tribute to a strong, courageous and inspiring woman," said Ontario MP John McKay.

The Members of Parliament stood and cheered.

Afterwards, Barb called me up. Never had there been such excitement in her voice. "It was an incredible room," she said of her morning talk. "It was kids who were totally silent and the moment was probably, well, I feel it was my most powerful presentation I've ever done. The kids stood up, and the tears, and the standing ovation. It was just phenomenal human beings."

The Prime Minister shook her hand, Barb said.

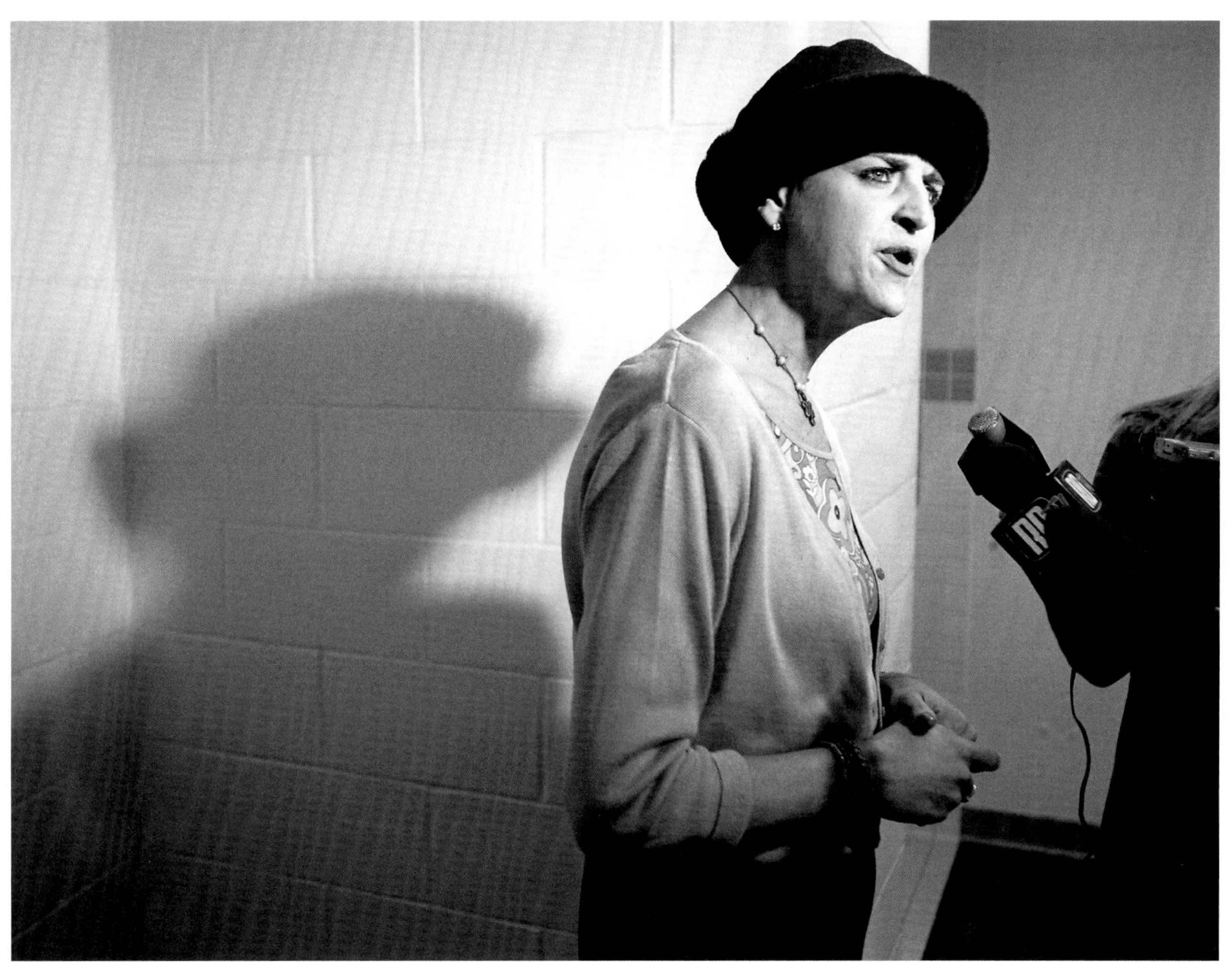

Barb talks to the media after her speech in Red Deer.

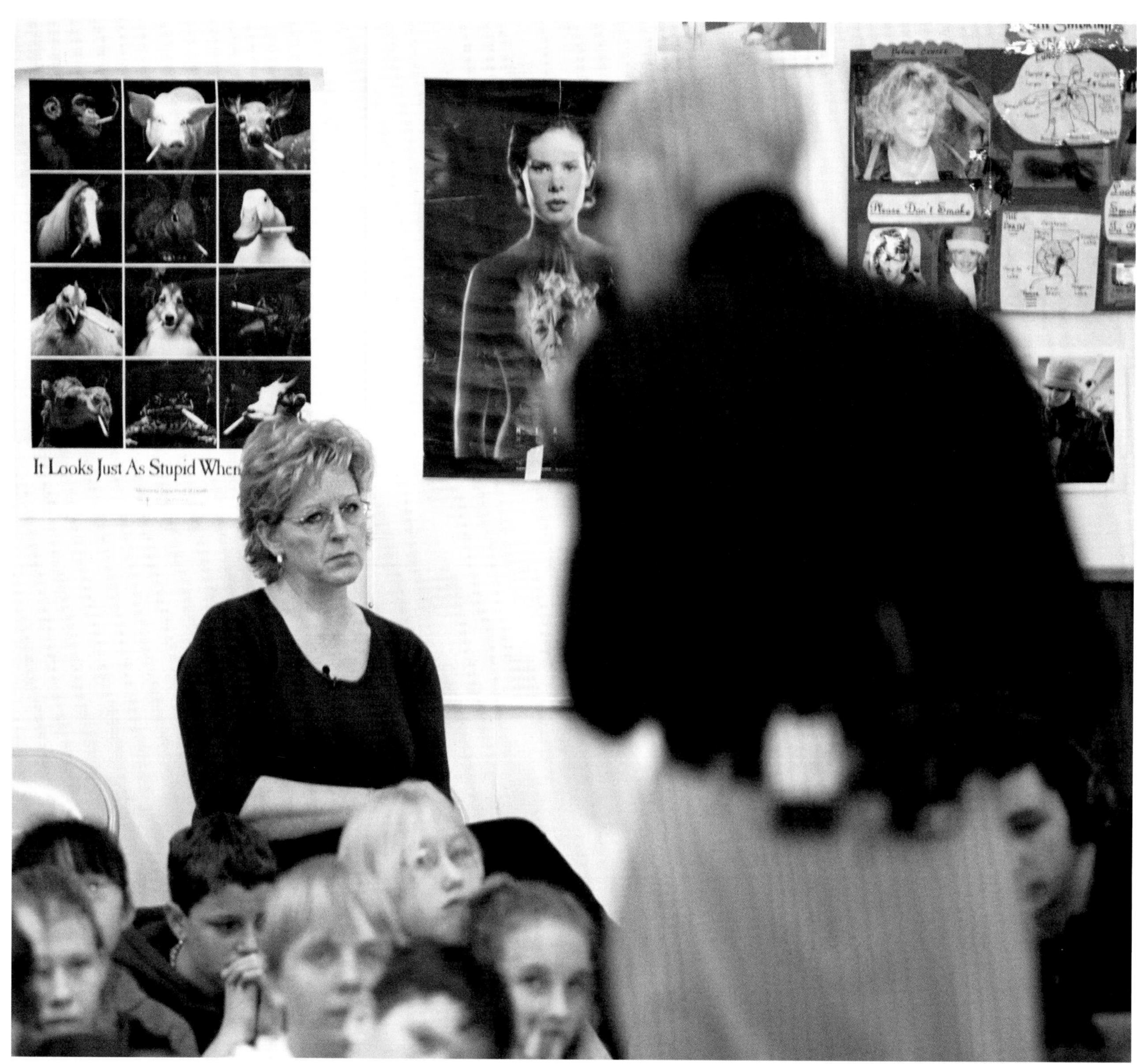

Tracy sits through another one of Barb's talks.

"He thanked me for the work I am doing for Canadians. I just said that this is what life is all about. I'm so full of energy right now that I could run a marathon."

As for the standing ovation, she said: "I got to tell you, sweetie, it was the most overwhelming experience of my life. I can't even begin to explain how I feel. I didn't think this would go, and it did."

That night, Barb, Tracy and Craig caught a flight to Toronto for Barb's presentation the next day.

The success of her crusade in Ontario made it clear to me and my editors that a change of direction was needed. We had always planned to write one large story detailing the entirety of her crusade after she had died. Now, though, with her work suddenly taking on national significance, we decided we'd better write the story in two parts, one now, one after her death.

I had one concern, that what we published was going to put our relationship with Barb in jeopardy. Outside of a handful of nasty letters and phone calls, she had received only laudatory press coverage so far. In this story, I would be addressing her habit of downplaying how much she was still smoking and how tired and upset Tracy had become with her demands and the grinding schedule. There was a good chance that Barb would stop co-operating with us after publication, I believed.

Saturday, February 8. "I've seen anti-smoking ad campaigns from various provinces and the federal government and they're all pretty well done, but none of them affected me the way the Barb Tarbox story did," Dan Kearney of Halifax, Nova Scotia, wrote to Barb, saying he'd seen her story on the CBC *National.* "I'm not really sure why, but when I heard her tell the story of the boy who crumpled up his cigarettes and gave them to her, I was inconsolable. I immediately grabbed the half-finished pack that I had, crumpled it up, and threw it in the garbage. I also poured olive oil on them so that I couldn't try to piece them back together later on when I was feeling the need for nicotine. Today I went out and got the patch."

Sunday, February 9. Just back from their Red Deer-Ottawa-Toronto trip, Barb and Tracy were on an airplane again today, this time with me and Greg in tow. We were flying to Vancouver, where Barb would meet with film writer Robert French on a stop-over, then on to Victoria, where Barb was to speak.

I sat next to Tracy on the plane to debrief her on the last leg of the crusade. I expected to find her as enthused as Barb, but I quickly discovered that they'd never been so far apart.

The first night at the Chateau Laurier in Ottawa, she and Barb had shared a room, but Tracy said she'd hardly slept; Barb had cranked the heat as high as it could go. In Toronto, Tracy had to get her own room to get away from the smoke, the heat, the tension.

She'd seen Barb speak 34 times now, Tracy said, the same basic speech. She knew when Barb would move her hands, when she'd weep, when she'd shout, everything she'd say. "I'm becoming bored with it. . . Whereas Barb gets pumped up and excited each morning, I just go, 'Aw shit.'"

At the Ottawa talk, which Barb had considered to be her best yet, Tracy said she felt embarrassed because Barb was so out-of-control angry. She was

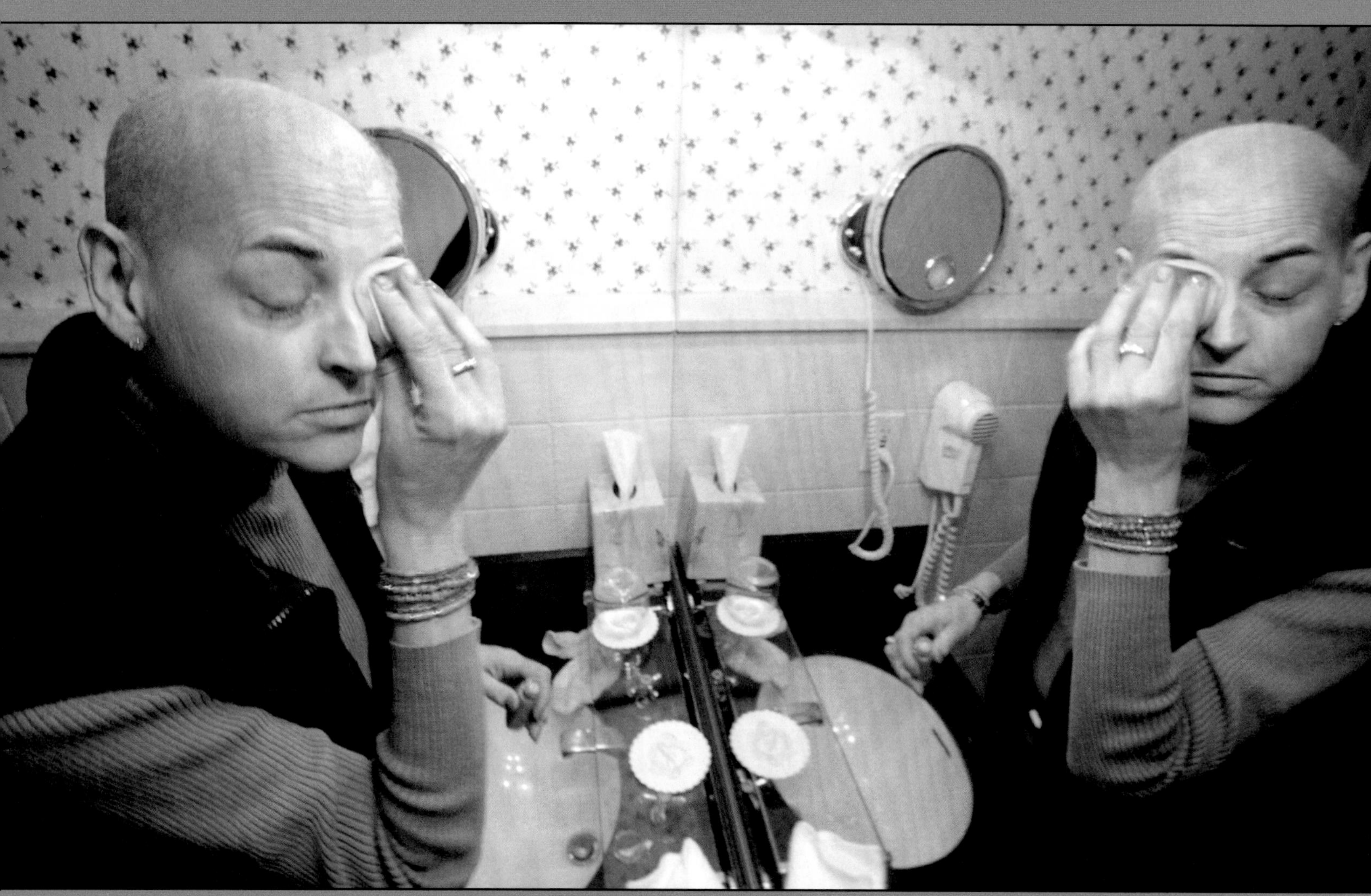

Barb applies makeup at 6 a.m. as she often has trouble sleeping. She wore stage makeup that often took up to an hour to apply.

so busy talking about her pain, Tracy said, that at times she forgot to mention smoking. "When you're winging your hat off and stomping your feet, these things just make the kids think she's psycho."

Tracy had suggested to Barb after the visit to the House of Commons that Barb should take her own advice about smoking, and instead of going out for a smoke, they should go out for a walk and take some pictures of the Peace Tower. It would be her only chance to get such photographs, Tracy told Barb. Barb had scoffed at the suggestion, desperate as she was to be in private for a smoke.

Several times, Barb broke down crying, Tracy said, likely because of the tension. Barb had also complained about her medication and how it was changing her personality. "I told her, 'I'm going to agree with you there. Your personality has been affected. Don't take offence here, but you're not the friend I knew two months ago. You're totally obsessed with the media, and I can't stand it. You seem to have no respect for my work and my family. This is not my story and my legacy. I'm just behind you and it's too late to back out.' "

Barb's smoking fibs continued to grate. In Ottawa, Barb had told a CBC reporter she was down to one a day when, in fact, she smoked steadily through the day. Tracy said she confronted Barb on this, but got nowhere. In restaurants, though, when someone walked past, Barb would try to hide her cigarette. "She doesn't want anything tarnished. As a friend I think I should tell her, 'Don't be lying. Be consistent with your stories.' People shouldn't think of her as a saint. She has her flaws."

Tracy told me she didn't know what to believe with Barb any more.

Tracy's husband Werner had been planning to go back to work all through January, but had stayed home to help her and the kids, because she was helping Barb. Their daughter Miranda was sick with the flu. Their other daughter Tiffany needed a tooth pulled. Tracy felt guilty. "It's like looking after another child that is taking up all your time and you're leaving the other two out."

Tracy, too, said she wasn't well, that she'd been having chest pains.

When Tracy arrived home on Saturday, she'd had to go into the office and work 13 hours. When she got back from this Vancouver/Victoria trip on Monday night, she knew she would have to go in to work.

Barb had wanted to book three more trips to Calgary, but Tracy told her she couldn't go, that she was needed at work and at home, that her kids were starting to suffer.

I asked Tracy why she didn't just bow out for a time.

"I have to keep going," she said. "I have no choice, I think. I'm major involved in this. If I won't do anything, she won't."

There was something inevitable about what she was doing here, something fated, Tracy told me. "I'm a Capricorn. We're very loyal and we're committed to everything we take on. I feel extremely loyal to Barb and extremely committed. But I do want to get back to normal."

A moment later, Tracy added: "I'm sure I get on her nerves, too."

When we got into Vancouver, Barb was sulking. She told us she was going to cancel her meeting with Robert French and just stay at the airport. We should go into Vancouver, she said, have fun. She'd be fine, even if our connecting flight wasn't for six hours. I suspected she had overhead Tracy and me.

After some effort, we persuaded Barb to meet with French. He came to the airport and took us into the city in his van.

Clouds and mist made the sky grey. Winter hung on across Canada, but spring reigned here, no snow, cool and rainy, lots of green.

"Look at the beautiful trees," Barb said. "I love this. And look at the size of that hedge!"

She had never expected to see spring again, but here it was, and Barb revelled in it for the moment. She hadn't been in this city for 19 years, she said, not since 1982, when she got the call that her mom had cancer and needed her.

French was a quiet fellow who came across more as an accountant than a movie man, but Barb quickly took to his soft-spoken manner. As we drove, she listed her symptoms for him, including one that was new to me: she'd bought three new kinds of mascara, then realized the problem wasn't the make-up, it was that her eyelids were shriveling.

She told French that she realized her mood was changing for the worse: "I was always phenomenally patient. I'm not now. I know it. I'm not blind. This is what it does and it's going to get worse. You can't ignore it. You can't pretend."

She used to work with disabled children, she said, and had to be patient. Now her irritable spells overwhelmed her. "In Ottawa, I went six and a half hours without a smoke. That's when I get irritable. I'm like, *I want it now!*

"The cancer is touching every part of me," she continued. "But you know what? I'm fighting all the way to my last breath. I'm going to say to the cancer, 'You can't touch my spirit, and you can't touch my soul.' I'm going to be the most stubborn cancer patient there ever was."

Barb rolled down the window and breathed in. "God, did I want this."

She pointed out an old apartment building where she had once lived. "The good-byes," she said softly.

We searched for a restaurant on Denman. Barb wanted a fish place.

"Can you smoke here?" she asked French.

"No."

"Except in lounges?"

"No, not even in the lounge," he said, then told Barb about Vancouver's restrictive new anti-smoking rules.

At lunch, French and Barb discussed the film project. If a movie was to be made, he said, they needed to broaden the story so it would appeal to at least a million viewers.

"I'm going insane here trying to get the high numbers of kids," Barb said of her own quest. "I'm a firm believer that right now I've been given extra time. It's for a reason. I'm not questioning. I still feel there is something more I have to accomplish, and I hope I will. Doctors can't explain it. They don't know where the strength comes from."

French told Barb he was certain her story had reach. "Here's a story that is going to move people and in a magical way. Like the Terry Fox story, it's a tragic story, but something positive is coming out of it. It's so rare."

He'd lost his own stepfather to cancer, French said.

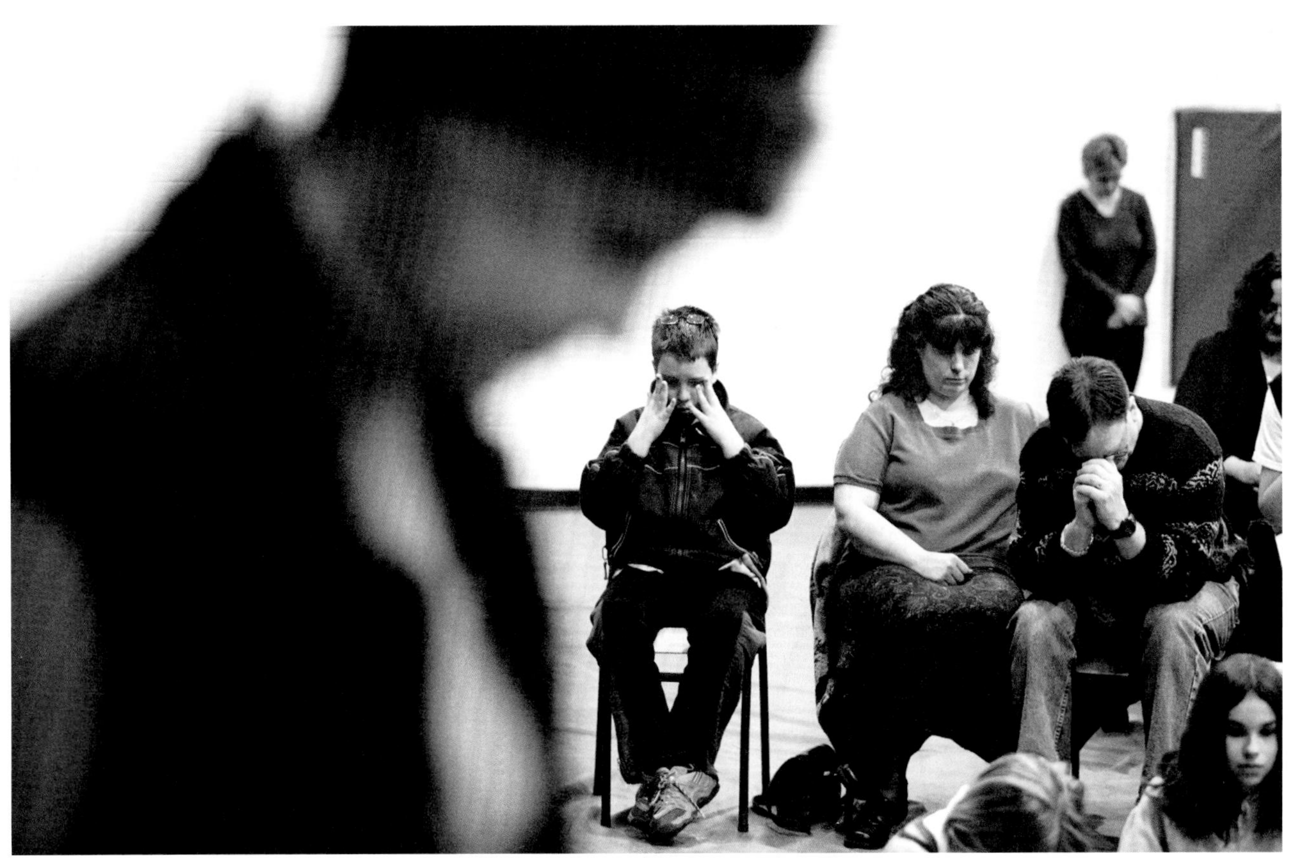

Barb bows her head in prayer after one of her talks in Victoria. Her brother Wes (bent over) and his family had come to hear her speak.

Back then, cancer was hush-hush. No one in his family was allowed to talk about his dad being sick. His parents believed in faith healing, but when it wasn't happening, everyone went into denial about the disease. French said he found the silence to be shameful and humiliating.

He told Barb he wouldn't stick to her story exactly, but would use elements of it, maybe use something from the CBC documentary where Barb had talked about meeting with young Luc Caouette in Leduc, and how he'd reminded her of Michael.

"I see him as representing teen smokers," French said.

One scene would show Barb early on in her illness, watching and doing nothing as some kids got older teens to buy them cigarettes. "It's a conspiracy of silence that causes so much of our trouble," French said, still evidently smarting from the silences of his own childhood home. "I want this story to be as raw and honest as you can."

"You got to be honest," Barb said, and added she always told the kids she was a smoker. "I'm not going to lie to them."

After lunch, Barb walked for a moment on the beach at English Bay, looking out into the distance at the birds, ships and sea. We then got a cab to head back to the airport.

"Are we allowed to smoke in your cab?" Barb asked the driver.

He gave no answer, but had a "No Smoking" sign up. Barb accepted his silence as a negative.

"It should be this way," she said quietly. "It should be."

Still, she schemed, saying she was going to find a smoking lounge at the airport. "I can sit. I can relax. I can smoke," she said and smiled. "It doesn't take a lot to get a wee bit excited."

Barb turned to Tracy. "I hope when I get to heaven there's a smoking lounge."

We all laughed.

We found one place at the Vancouver airport, a cafeteria-style bar, the Stanley Lounge, that allowed smoking. I sat down with Barb, and decided it was time to go over some of the controversial issues. I had to get her side of things for my story.

I first asked Barb why she didn't buy her own cigarettes, but had Tracy do it. She told me she didn't want to go into her old convenience store any more, the place she'd bought smokes for years. "They're so kind, and they have been for years. I don't want to see the pain in their eyes."

She didn't want others to know how much she smoked, she said. "Think about it. I'm flippin' bald, and I'm saying, 'Could I have a pack of cigarettes?' It is embarrassing because I'm still addicted."

Next, I asked her about being obsessed with her crusade, and, in Tracy's eyes, with the media.

"I've developed friendships with the media," she said, listing off Al Stafford from CHED, Serena Mah from CFRN-TV, and Leslie Macdonald from Global TV. "It's hard for others to understand that. I have media within the city that call me just to say hi. I know I spend too much time talking to them. But I like the kids, the teachers, the media."

So far, she'd missed very little time with Mackenzie or Pat because of her speaking, she said. This was the first weekend she was away, she said, and part of it was to see her brother, Wes, and his family in Victoria.

But Barb said she could understand Tracy's upset. "She's the most phenomenal gifted worker you'll ever meet in your life. But she's tired."

On the plane to Victoria, Barb and Tracy sat together. Barb warned Tracy to be careful about the things she was telling me: "David can twist things you say."

Tracy wondered why Barb was being so defensive. If Barb always told the truth, there would be nothing for her to worry about, Tracy thought.

Still, by the time the two got off the plane, they were laughing. They'd been looking at a man and a woman on the plane and speculating about the two of them having an affair.

Barb was also buoyant because she'd at last convinced herself it was time to let Greg take a picture of her without any make-up. The photo shoot was planned for early the next morning in her hotel room.

Barb's brother Wes and his wife, also named Tracy, met us at the airport. Wes was a local bus driver, and seemed the opposite of Barb: quiet, husky, introverted.

It was dark out, cool but not raining. Wes and Tracy took us in their van to the old Royal Empress Hotel on the bay. After a quiet supper, we retreated to our rooms to prepare for another hectic day.

Monday, February 10. A second e-mail came in for Barb from Joan Dundas of Brock University. When she used to take cigarette breaks, she said she'd always been joined by a student, Mohammed. "The week after I saw your broadcast (on the CBC), I told him that he was welcome to go for a cigarette outside, but that I wouldn't be joining him. Of course, he was curious."

Dundas said she took him to the computer, and they watched the CBC documentary on Barb on the Internet. "The next week, he informed me he had also quit smoking."

In the morning, Barb kept her promise. Greg came in with his cameras and took pictures of her before she applied her make-up. A roadmap of upraised veins covered her lower body. Greg thought her face didn't look all that different without the make-up, though Barb's vanity was surely telling her otherwise. She dressed in her usual spiffy fashion, wearing a green hat, black turtleneck sweater and black leather skirt. Wes came to pick us up for the school presentation. We exited the hotel to see cherry trees blossoming all around. Today, though, spring wasn't enough to rejuvenate Barb. Her breathing sounded laboured.

"OK, guys," she said. "My knees aren't working today."

"Where's your cane?" Wes asked.

"It's at home. You know what? I should have brought it. I'm totally off balance and I can really feel it."

Pacific Christian school had 550 students in its gym to hear Barb. As Tracy and Barb prepared for the talk, I took a moment to speak to Wes about his little sister.

Barb had always been a talker, he said. "She's never had a problem with shyness. She was never afraid to say what was on her mind."

Her anger erupted repeatedly during the talk. In parts where she'd been quiet and weepy before, such as when she talked about saying goodbye to her friends and family, she now raged. "If anybody ever says that smoking only affects you and nobody else, think again! *Think again!* You tell me how cool it is to bury somebody you love."

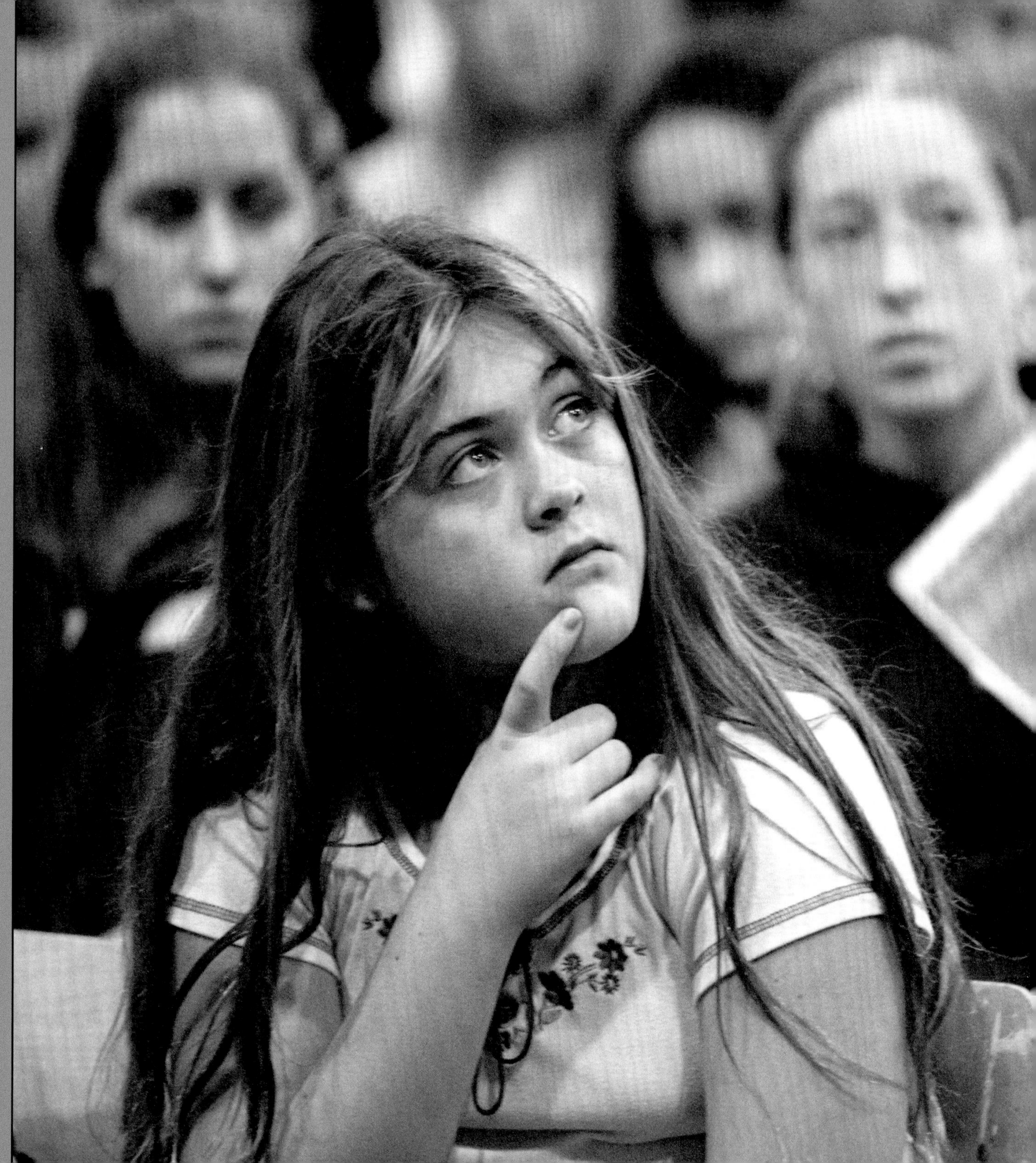

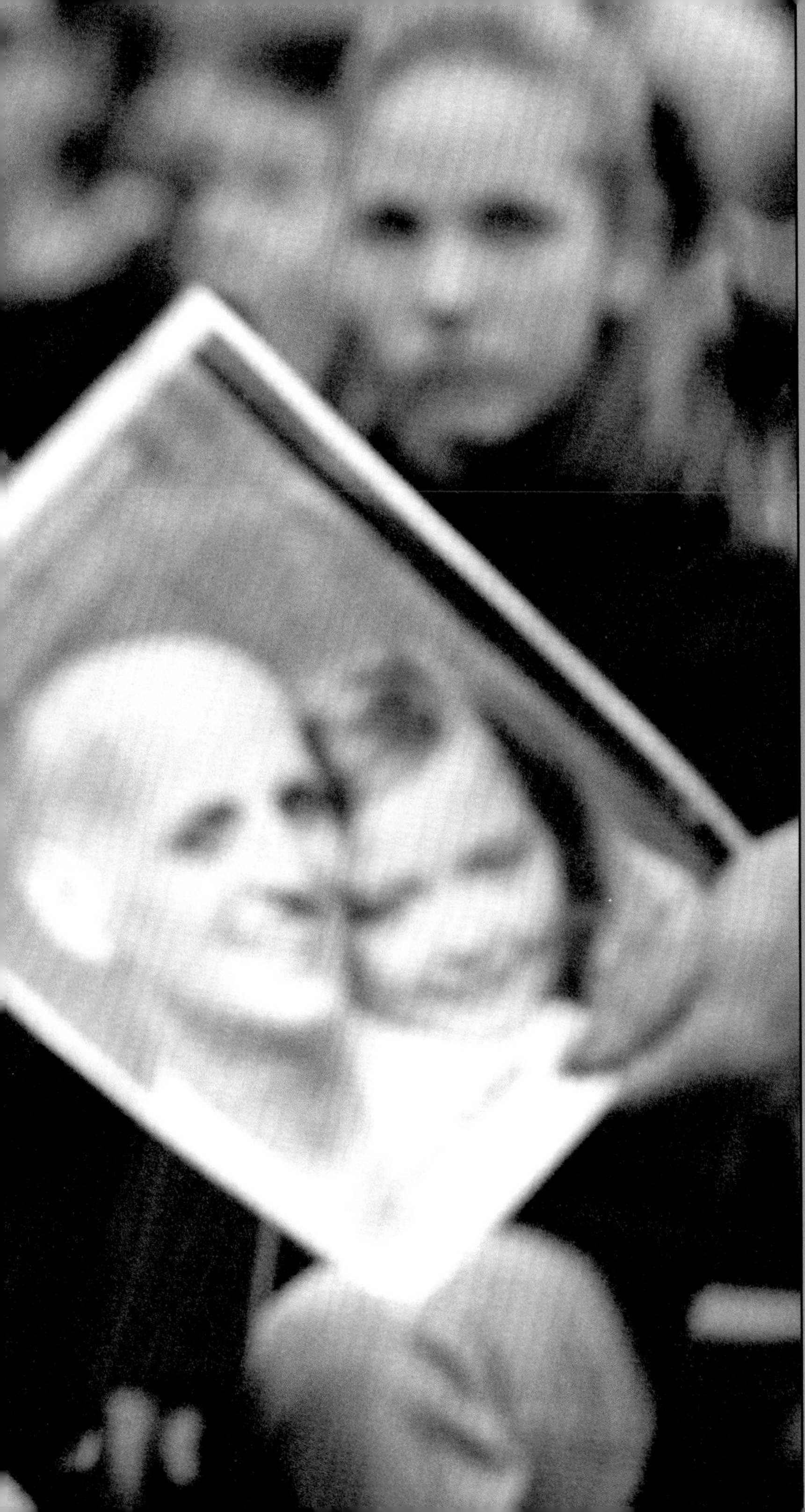

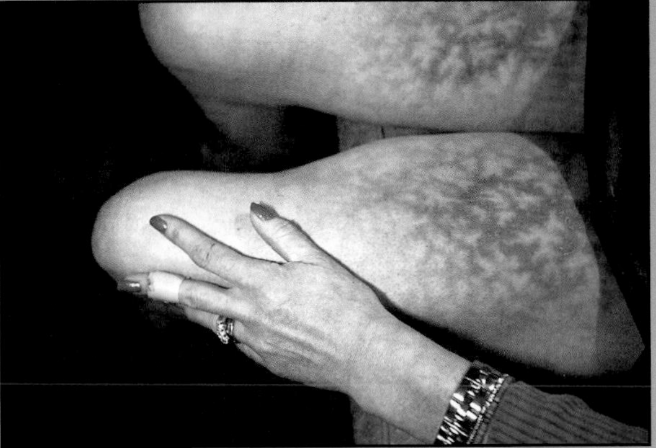

As a result of the cancer, the veins in Barb's legs are black and elevated.

Students in Victoria listen to Barb speak as she holds a picture of herself and Mackenzie, just one of many pictures she used in her presentations.

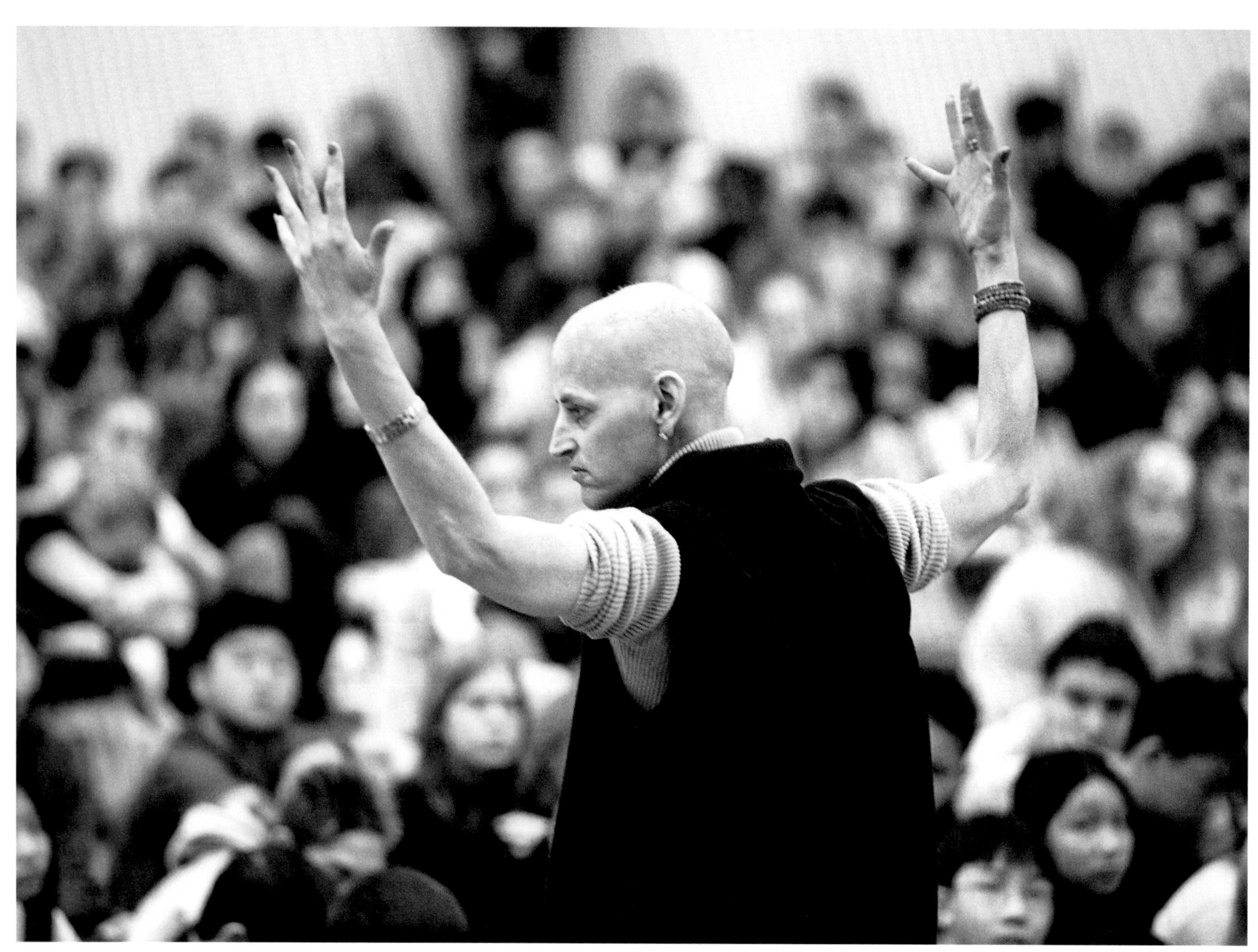

Barb rolls up her sleeves during one of her speeches to allow students to see her withering body.

She told the kids she owned 60 pairs of shoes but her feet were now so swollen she could only wear one of those pairs.

After her talk, the school principal asked the kids to pray for her. "She has a heart for other people so let us have a heart for her," said David O'Dell.

Barb's energy boost from her talk was short-lived. Dozens of kids wanted to hug her. One young girl suggested to Barb it would be OK for her to die, since she would go to heaven and see Jesus and all her loved ones who had died before. Barb told the girl that God's plan for people included them being good spouses and good parents, and her death would stop her from doing that.

After a short time, Barb made to leave. "That's enough, kids," she said

It was the first time she'd departed so quickly. Pressure had built up in her chest, squeezing her. In the van, heading to the airport, she looked ashen. "Oh, I'm frozen," she said. "I was feeling overwhelmed. I thought I was going to drop."

"That would add dramatic flair," Wes said.

"No teasing, Wes," Tracy said from the backseat. "You won't be able to watch any more talks if you're going to tease."

At the airport, Barb didn't say good-bye to Wes, just that she'd see him again, at the end of March, when she again planned to come out here again to speak.

On the plane, she collapsed into her seat. She'd pushed Tracy to the edge, and now she'd done the same to herself.

"I'm tired," she said. "Just tired."

I knew what she meant. I'd only been on the road for two days, and I wasn't sick with cancer, but I felt exhausted. Barb and Tracy had been traveling for almost a week now, but still had out-of-town talks planned for the next two days.

Tuesday, February 11. "What Terry Fox is to cancer research, Barb Tarbox is to cancer prevention," wrote Ian Hunter of Kanata in a letter in the *Ottawa Citizen*. "Both are true Canadian heroes."

Barb got another e-mail from Breanne Fisher from Ottewell school. She'd done a study, she said. Of the 44 students in grades seven, eight and nine that used to smoke, 26 said they had now quit. "Wow, you have saved so many lives!"

Barb and Tracy headed off for a presentation in Camrose, an hour outside the city. I went to work on my major story, which was to run on Sunday. In the piece, I needed to address how successful Barb's crusade had been. There was no way of knowing exactly how many people had quit smoking because of her, but I was curious to see if Luc Caouette, the Leduc teenager, had been able to stay off cigarettes. I got him on the phone.

"I'm doing pretty good," he said. "I'm on some medication to quit. It stops *the nic* from happening, so I'm down to about one smoke a day."

I asked him what he meant by *the nic*. He said it was his craving for a smoke. "When I'm *niccing*, it's like I'm missing something from me. I need the cigarette, to be complete."

I asked him about Barb.

"I think she is a good lady."

He asked if Barb was still alive and was relieved to hear she was.

"She made a big impact on my life. I think in the future, in many years, she should become a saint. She saved my life."

Wednesday, February 12. Barb and Tracy flew to the northern Alberta city of Grande Prairie, where Barb spoke to 4,000 students. Afterwards, Ava Dales, the local woman who organized the talk, sent Tracy a note. "There are no words that could possibly convey the way Barb touched our community. The buzz here is deafening. Give my best and my best to you, too, Tracy. You rock."

Later that day, when Barb had returned home, I called her with the good news about Luc Caouette.

"Oh my God!" she gushed. "There's something about that kid. But, you know, I don't think I'm a saint. No way at all. I'm just grateful. All I've wanted was for one person to throw away the cigarettes and for every additional one that does it, I feel incredibly blessed. I feel blessed for them, and for their families, and the people that love them. There is no pain worse than grief."

She had buried her own parents and her twins, she reminded me. "That pain is phenomenal. And now all the arrangements are made for my death. So I need to do this. I *need* to do this. I don't know the reason. . . But you know what? I am still so incredibly serious. I am doing this until my last breath. I am not stopping."

I pointed out to Barb that while Tracy had complaints about her, she never complained about Tracy, or about Pat.

"That's not the way I've ever been," she said. "Tracy will get tired when I've taken on too much. . . We're women. We can get stubborn with each other for five minutes, and then it's done. We don't worry about it. Without her, I can't have done all of this. We're nutty at the best of times, we're serious at the best of times, and we're emotional, that's us, that's how we will always be."

Thursday, February 13. Barb sent me a note, asking that in the story I put in a huge thanks to Tracy's employer, Team Ford. "If it wasn't for them, this wouldn't be possible. I think this is the most incredible company."

She also mentioned that the Montel Williams show in New York was now talking about doing a special on her.

Friday, February 14. Carol Wiebe of St. Albert e-mailed Barb to say she'd been smoking for 27 years, since she was in grade seven. She was a single mother of two young girls, and for many years they'd been after her to quit. One evening this past January, Wiebe had been on her way out to the garage for a smoke, when she went to turn off the TV. Just then, one of Barb's AADAC ads came on. "It felt like you were talking directly to me. It was such a wake-up call. . . God bless and peace be with you."

Sunday, February 16. The *Journal* story, "To Her Last Breath," came out, a 9,000-word report over six pages, with 18 of Greg's photographs, including shots of Barb smoking and without her make-up. Tracy e-mailed Greg and me that afternoon. She'd already gotten an e-mail from Ava Dales, the Grande Prairie organizer, who had raved about how great the article was. Tracy told us the story brought back so many things she'd forgotten. "I really like the story, except of course the parts where Barb and I are fighting. Mind you, no one likes to read they are not perfect. I haven't been able to get a hold of Barb, so I'm thinking she is pissed at me. I left two phone messages and two e-mails telling her to contact me. So we will have to see."

Monday, February 17. In the morning, Barb e-mailed her volunteer helper Donna Gingera about the story, but not Tracy. "I experienced the most judgmental, critical statements that I have ever in my life," Barb said. "I had no idea Tracy was bored with the presentations and that she didn't want to be there any more with me. I did not know this and I do apologize. I will not ask any further assistance as of this moment, immediately.

"Reading in the *Edmonton Journal* what an impatient and nasty human being I am was really the icing on the cake. I had no idea that the *Edmonton Journal* and Tracy felt so strong about this. It is very obvious the documentary is now completed. . . There will be no Part 2 in this and I believe that to be how it should be now. The moment of my death is something I take very personally and I would not want my moment of the last breath to be abused with everything I do wrong. I thank you all for all the work you have done in the past and I wish you much happiness. Barb."

At the same time as Barb fumed, Pat was telling her to calm down. "You know what, they have to tell the whole story, Barb," he said. "It's not like this editorial is on the sainthood of Barb Tarbox. You have to understand that Tracy is getting a little frustrated and David asked her about it, and David is being honest and so is Tracy. Don't get mad at them."

Barb's hurt didn't surprise me. I'd been a newspaper columnist for many years, and had been the target of many angry letter writers; I understood how it stung to get criticized. I hoped her upset would pass. I was sure I'd been fair to her. Still, whenever I thought that our work with her might be over, sadness welled up in me.

Greg's emotions were more mixed. A part of him felt relief. Unlike me, his job doesn't encourage him to be aloof. Instead, it is up to him to get as close as possible to his subjects. Through his lens, he was always in Barb's face. He needed her permission, her friendship, to get that close.

On the Victoria trip, Greg noticed huge physical changes in Barb, and he knew it was only going to get worse. The stress of his proximity was starting to overwhelm him. When he read Barb's upset note, it occurred to him that maybe it was best for everyone to pull back. Barb could move away from the media spotlight and be alone with her family. He could get on with his normal life and avoid getting an ulcer.

Another part of him, though, felt terrible that he might not be able to do the work that both he and Barb had agreed was so important.

Donna forwarded Barb's e-mail to Tracy. Tracy replied directly to Barb. "Let's talk about this article . . . It shouldn't have been assumed that David was going to paint a rosy picture on everything because it is not rosy. You know that, I know that, everyone else who has had a dear one suffer with cancer knows that. . . You are considered as being a saint, and we all, David, Greg, Craig and even Donna think you are absolutely amazing, and I know you can feel that from us. David,

Greg and mostly me want to be part of your life . . . If you choose to shut me out with the rest of them, then I will start to question our level of friendship. I always thought it went way, way beyond that."

Tuesday, February 18. In the morning, Tracy broke down at work and wept in the women's bathroom over her fight with Barb. Part of her felt like a very bad friend.

For her part, Barb's feelings were changing. The inbox of her e-mail was now full of messages complimenting both her work and the *Journal* story. Still, she was upset with Tracy, and uncertain about how Tracy really felt about her.

She e-mailed Tracy late in the afternoon: "I still believe you are my best friend, and I wish all your dreams to come true. I can only hope now that life finishes quickly for me because we have always said life makes us laugh. Please say prayers now for my death because I just want you to be happy in life. It's amazing how comments to one writer has peeled us (apart). And we allowed it. Barb."

In response, Tracy wrote to Barb that she had no intention of cutting her out of her life. "Honestly, I will fight to get back into your life. When you said in your last e-mail, 'Pray for my death now,' yes, I felt like shit. I don't think one writer has pulled us apart. I think it goes deeper. But you have to realize this is your life, and I'm very happy all this happened for you. You deserve everything good that comes out of this. This is not what my life is about, and I'm sorry I can't be as passionate and excited as you with this all. Do you think we can still go to Montreal or is your physical situation too bad?"

When Tracy showed me her note to Barb, I was grateful. She could have sold me out, as Barb was evidently ready to do, but she had stood up for me. I admired her integrity. If we hadn't been friends before, we were now.

Wednesday, February 19. Barb again contacted Tracy, saying she was ready to go to Montreal next week and wasn't going without Tracy. But just as this internal feud was ending, another outside controversy had started up. In the day's paper, *Journal* editors ran parts of a letter that had been sent to me by Rand Wakeford, a local man known for his work as a Society for the Prevention of Cruelty to Animals officer.

"Barb Tarbox is NOT a hero," Wakeford said. "Barb Tarbox does not shun the cancerous weapons that have left her and her family ravaged and wrecked. Barb Tarbox takes time out of her day to lovingly caress that weapon. To soulfully place that weapon to her lips like a long lost lover, to inhale the poisonous smoke that caresses her lungs like a serpent. Barb Tarbox says that her doctor says it's too late to quit now. Get real Barb. Get a new doctor. Get a life. Oops, sorry, too late for that, too."

Thursday, February 20. AADAC officials and several Tory MLAs invited Barb to the Alberta Legislature. AADAC was set to announce the Barb Tarbox Awards of Excellence in Tobacco Reduction and an annual scholarship in her name.

At the Legislature, the MLAs stood to give Barb an ovation. Barb, Tracy, Greg and I then went to a private area downstairs, where other MLAs talked to Barb. To help her with travel expenses, and in recognition of her work, an AADAC official gave her a $12,000 cheque.

Barb hadn't asked for this payment. "This is phenomenal," she said. "I'm totally speechless. I'd cry, but the make-up would go all over the place."

"We've got to go to New York now!" Tracy said.

The four of us then went to lunch at Earl's Tin Palace, an upscale burger joint. During her Legislature appearance, a group of firefighters in the upper gallery had stood up and cheered for Barb, though they'd been instructed by security staff not to leave their seats. Barb loved it.

"I'm bald and I can still get a man in trouble," she said, and we all laughed.

It was good to be together as a group again, but I still felt shaky with Barb. I no longer fully trusted her commitment to us and to the project, and was ready to walk away from it if that's what Barb wanted. I told Barb I needed to hear that she really wanted us to document her last weeks. She said she did.

In the evening, Tracy sent me an e-mail. "Well, that was fun today, don't you think? I guess there will be Part Two. I think Barb is OK with everything now. I think she might actually be relieved that she doesn't have to portray she's perfect anymore to the public, and that even while they know that, they still love her."

Friday, February 21. Despite the vitriol of letter writer Rand Wakeford's attack on Barb, and anything negative that came out in my article, the public's affection for Barb only grew.

Letters flooded into the *Journal.* "Rand Wakeford says Barb Tarbox is not a hero because she still smokes," Ken Neilson of Edmonton wrote. "If I don't misunderstand her, I'd say Barb Tarbox probably agrees with this less-than-generous assessment. . . I believe the last thing she wants is for anyone to think of her as a role model. Rather, she has cast herself very much as the anti-hero, someone not to be emulated."

And Joan Fedio: "As a long term smoker who just stopped on Jan. 2, I can say that the last 49 days have been the longest and seemingly the most horrible days of my life. To insist that Ms. Tarbox go through that process to gain credibility with people like Rand Wakeford is ridiculous."

And B.C. Whitten: "Barb Tarbox is not a hypocrite. She's addicted. . . I'm not defending her because I'm a smoker. I am not. I'm just being reasonable. Try it."

And Carl Bergstrom: "A real hero is one who recognizes heroism in someone else, and Barb Tarbox by her crusade, recognizes the possibility of heroism in the young."

Monday, February 24. Barb and Tracy flew to Montreal. They had planned to go shopping, but after walking a few blocks, Barb said she was too tired to continue. She was eating, though, three or four chocolate bars for supper and a couple bags of chips. She and Tracy stayed up late, talking until 11:30 p.m.

Tuesday, February 25. Barb got up at 4 a.m. in anticipation of her presentation to 1,200 students at Lower Canada College, her 38th in four months.

During her talk, Barb realized something was wrong. Her speech was so slurred that she feared the students might think she'd been drinking.

Tracy noticed Barb wasn't angry, like before, just confused. When she held up Tracy's picture to say

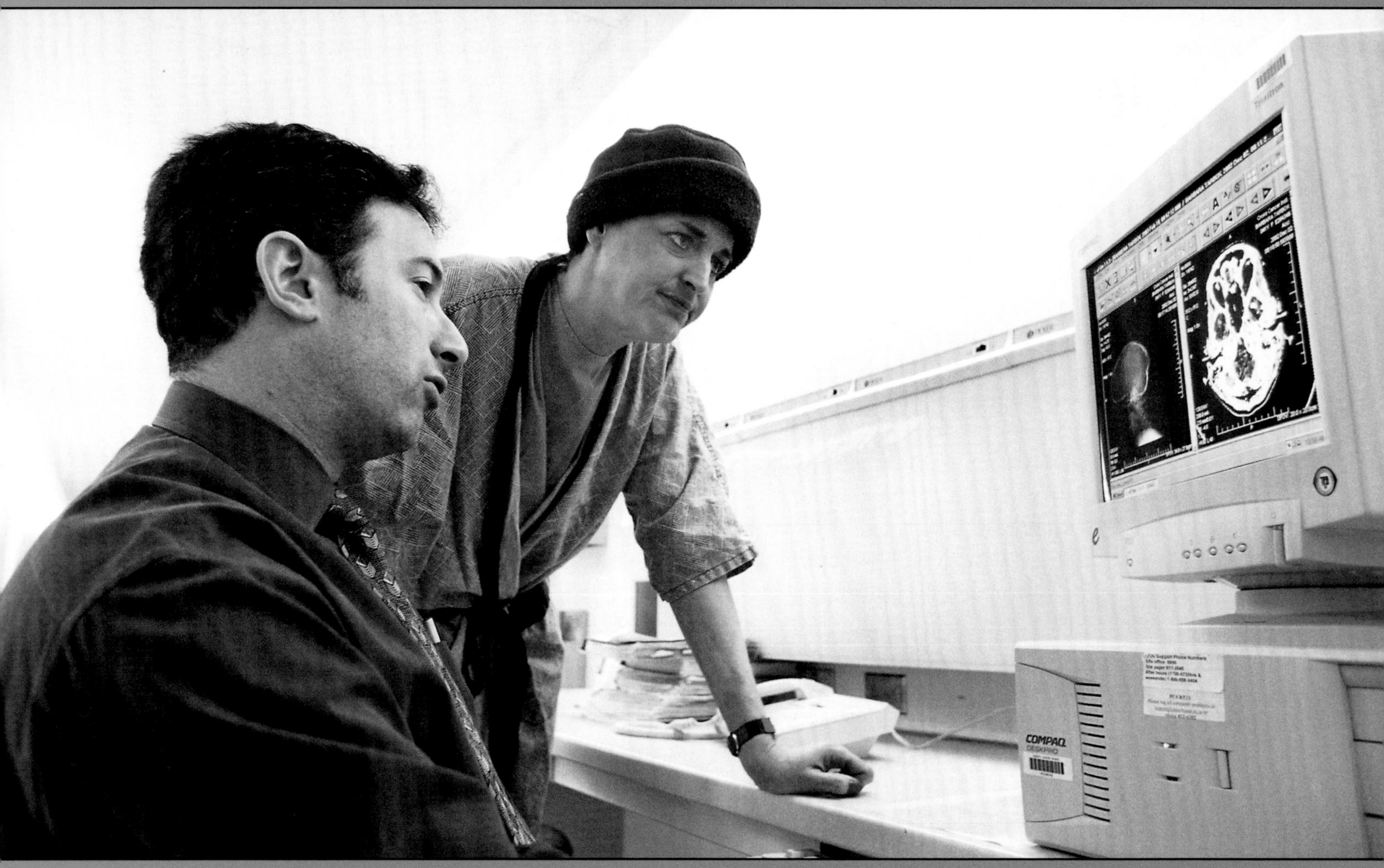

Dr. Ross Halperin shows Barb a CT scan of her brain which displays that the tumour has spread.

how much she was going to miss her, she got Tracy's name wrong. Next, Barb told the kids she faced the agony of burying Pat and Mackenzie, instead of them burying her. She repeated herself continually. Tracy ran the slide show, and had to put up images on the screen to prod Barb to talk about a new topic.

Afterwards, Barb felt no post-presentation euphoria, just tired and dizzy. At the airport, she bumped into walls. She kept digging her finger into her pill box, but when Tracy checked, she found Barb had missed taking at least one day's worth of her anti-seizure medications.

In the departure area, a woman recognized Barb, then told Barb about her father, who had lived with lung cancer for 17 years due to the healing properties of asparagus. Barb listened intently, but on the airplane she asked Tracy, "What is asparagus?"

Tracy was astonished. In the in-flight magazine, she found a picture of asparagus and showed it to Barb.

As the flight went on, Barb lapsed in and out of delirium.

"Why are you doing this to me?" she kept asking Tracy. "Where are my arms? What did you do with them? And where did you put the mustard?"

"I don't have any mustard, Barb. Are you hungry and do you want a hot dog?"

Barb glared at Tracy and smiled calmly, but made no sense. Tracy felt helpless to the point of tears.

They arrived in Edmonton at just before midnight. Tracy wanted to take Barb to the hospital, but she insisted they go home. First, though, Barb asked if they could go get asparagus. It was late, Tracy said, and no stores would be open that would sell the vegetable.

Wednesday, February 26. "Very sorry about Barb's health," Liliane Luwaga of Bergen, Norway, e-mailed Tracy. "Let us pray."

First thing in the morning, Barb sent Pat out to get some asparagus. Next, Barb called up Tracy. "Well, I have asparagus. Do I just carve it up and eat it?"

"I don't think it's best if it's raw," Tracy replied. "You could try steaming it."

Barb did that and called back two hours later, saying she had eaten two full bunches of asparagus.

"Take it easy," Tracy said. "You'll get a stomach ache."

In the afternoon, a string of massive headaches confined Barb to her living room couch. When Tracy called to check, she heard something new in Barb's voice: despair.

After work that evening, Pat brought fast food home for Barb and Mackenzie. He found Barb on the couch, holding her head in her hands. Barb asked Mackenzie to go and get her the stapler. Mackenzie fetched it, put it on the coffee table.

"No, I need the stapler," Barb said, irritated.

"It's right in front of you, sweetie," Pat said.

"No, I'm hungry. I want the stapler."

Pat realized Barb was talking about the hamburger he'd bought her. She continued to mix up words, then bent over in agony, seized by another headache.

"That's it, we're going to the hospital," Pat said, expecting her to protest.

"No," Barb said quietly. "It's OK. I want to go."

At the Grey Nuns, Barb collapsed into a bed. Tracy rushed over to join Pat and Mackenzie at her side. Tracy feared this was it for Barb, but Pat was less anxious, and focused on the fact that Barb was exhausted and hadn't taken all of her pills. He left the worry to Barb, he liked to say. He was logical, the equivalent of the stoic *Star Trek* character Spock.

For five hours, Barb hardly moved in her bed, as blood work was done, and X-rays and a CT scan were taken. When at last she woke up, it was the middle of the night. Her doctor told her she wouldn't be going home.

"Yes I am! I am going right now."

"Sweetie, you're staying in," Pat told Barb. "We have to find out what's going on."

"Don't talk to me like that! I am leaving."

Tracy and Pat both understood Barb's reluctance to be hospitalized. Barb feared it meant not only an end to her crusade, but also to her life. She agreed to stay over only after she went outside with Tracy for a calming smoke.

Through the early morning hours, Barb remained confused. A doctor asked her what day and month it was.

"Fernand, zero, seven point nine seven three, point two seven forty," she replied.

Just then, Mackenzie turned to Tracy. "My mom is just mixed up with her words."

"You don't have to explain stuff to Tracy," Pat said. "She knows."

"I know, Dad," Mackenzie said. "I'm just trying to be strong."

"You don't have to be strong," Pat told his daughter. "You can just be 10 years old."

Thursday, February 27. Tracy took Barb from the Grey Nuns to the Cross Cancer Institute to talk over the results of her tests with Dr. Halperin. Barb had Tracy stop at Tim Horton's. Barb ordered three boxes of donuts.

"Are we hungry?" Tracy asked.

"Oh no, we got to get them for the nurses."

The CT scan showed Barb's brain now had multiple tumours. Halperin showed Barb the images on a computer screen.

"Ah, man, this is not good," she said, frowning.

"We're in trouble," he said. "We do have another option. We can do radiation again. The chances of it working aren't as good as the first time around. Our other option is to leave things be and let nature take its course."

"Is that death in two weeks? I'm probably close."

"I can never tell you. The only thing I know about the time is, I'll be wrong. I can tell you about the average person, that untreated cancer in a person's brain carries with it about a one-month-long prognosis. Treated, is it different? Maybe, maybe not, because it may not respond."

The treatments might tire her out and give her headaches, Halperin told Barb. There was also a chance the radiation would damage her brain.

"You know what, Dr. Halperin," Barb said just then. "Book it. Do it. Let's go for it."

Halperin left the room, leaving Tracy and Barb alone.

"So more radiation," Tracy said uncertainly.

"I'm kind of missing it," Barb said.

Tracy laughed. "You are the weirdest person I've ever met in my life."

Barb laughed too. "Maybe I'm warped, and I'm beginning to think so, but what I want to do right now is fry the daylights out of the brain again. That will give me a couple more weeks, and that's what I want."

Later, I talked to Barb about all that transpired. Only for a day or two had she really gotten down, she said. "I was like, 'Will it not leave me alone long enough for me to finish talking to the kids?' I was exhausted. I'd never been tired like that. I sat there and I said, 'Something is wrong. Something has gone wrong.'"

Pat was now in charge of her daily pill intake, she said. "He's amazing. He really is. He's right in there now. He's taken over now. That's my husband, through and through. He's in charge of everything. My boss man. He's very strict, but he's so darn cute about it. He's incredible and he always has been."

I also talked to Tracy. She was starting to feel panic over Barb, she said. For months, her whole life had been wrapped up in Barb and the crusade. She now felt paralyzed. "I won't go anywhere. I wouldn't go skiing with Werner. What if something happened? That would be awful."

She was also fearful about the future, *her* future this time. "When Barb is gone, what am I going to do?"

Friday, February 28. "In the past nine weeks, six of us have quit smoking," Kelly Jones of Leduc wrote to Barb. "When I first saw Barb on the news, I was turned off. I was in fear of what she had to say. But I started to get convicted in my spirit: 'What makes you different than her?'

"I'm proud to say today is Day 20 of not smoking. I smoked for 22 years, my husband 27 years. I am so grateful to Barb Tarbox and I feel she needs to know that her mission God has sent her on is being fulfilled. Here's the names of my friends who have quit smoking . . . Darryce, two months. Tracy, nine weeks. Nancy, eight weeks. Trudy, eight days. Grahame, eight days. Wayne, 20 days. Kelly, 20 days."

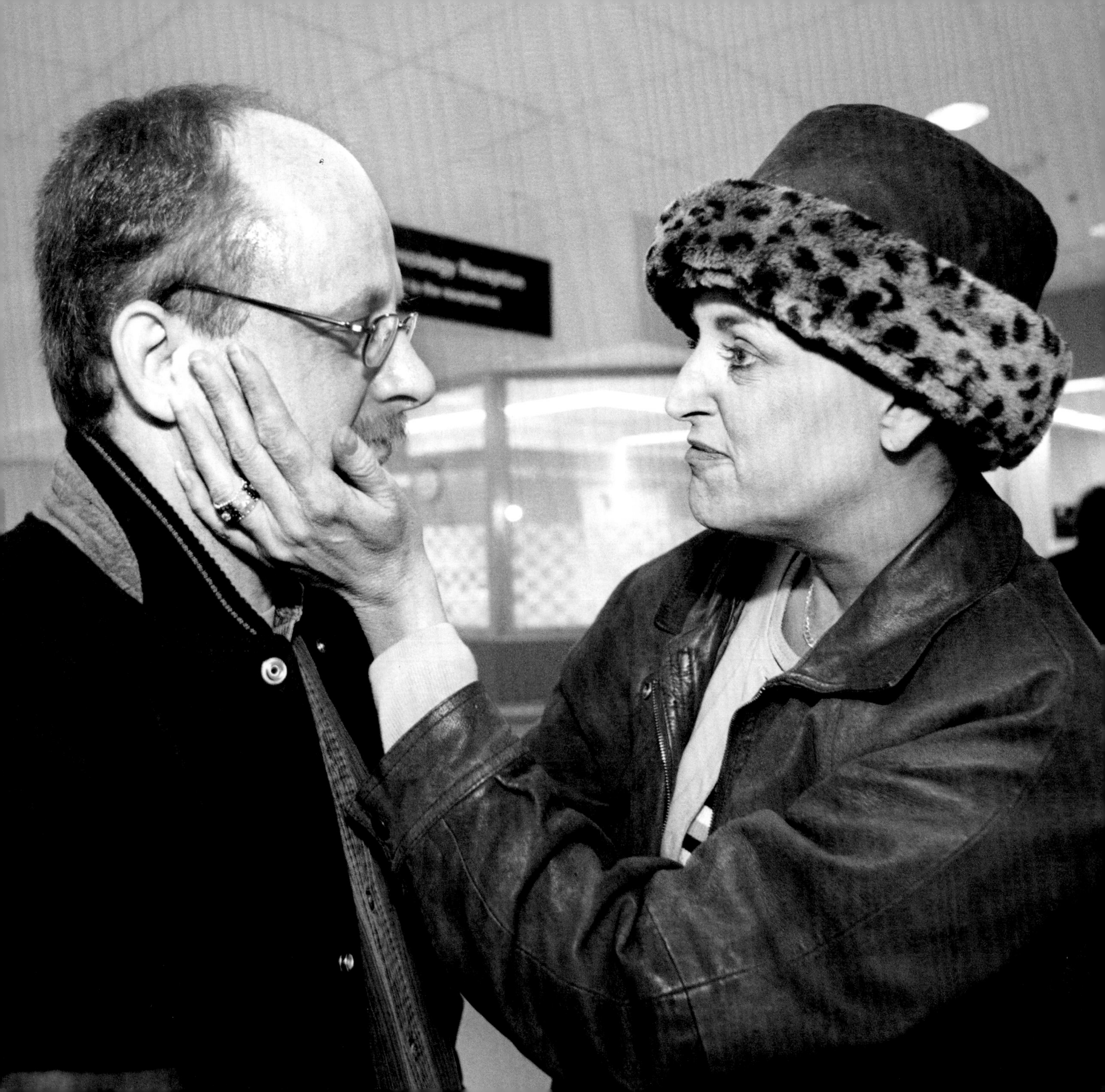

March

2 0 0 3

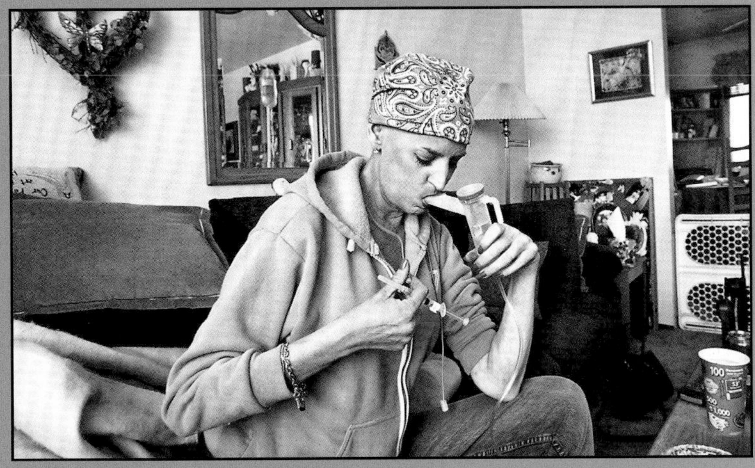

Distance does not make you falter,
now, arriving in magic, flying,
and finally, insane for the light,
you are the butterfly and you are gone

And so long as you haven't experienced
this: to die and so to grow,
you are only a troubled guest
on the dark earth.

Goethe
Translated by Robert Bly

Opposite page: Barb talks to Roy Trosin, a truck driver who heard Barb on the radio and gave up smoking.

Saturday, March 1. "I sit here in front of my computer, my first day without cigarettes, and I have you to thank for my strength," Carla Hilliard of Edmonton e-mailed Barb. "In the dark, weak moments of temptation, I play your 'good-bye' TV message over and over and over on my computer. Between tears running down my face and the fuzziness of my head right now, I can hardly type, but I know I will make it. . . . The Lord has given you a wonderful opportunity, and you have grasped it."

"What are we going to be doing today?" Mackenzie asked Barb in the morning.

"Mackenzie, could we just not have a day of stay-at-home?"

"Another one?" the girl whined.

At that, Barb exploded in anger.

Pat accepted Barb's moods. He explained to Mackenzie that Barb might be trying to push them away so they wouldn't love her so much, and they'd get used to her not being around.

Barb now had an explanation for her bad temper — her multiplying tumours — but her difficulties still frightened her. She struggled for calm. At home, she had always shoveled the walks, but now she had to rely on Pat. When he was slow to do the work, Barb bristled, stormed out and did it herself.

She started to unburden herself more and more to an old friend, her ex-sister-in-law, who by chance was also named Barb Tarbox. This Barb was divorced from Pat's younger brother Frank. To avoid confusion, everyone called her Little Barb, as she was just over five feet tall, compared with six-foot Barb. Little Barb was a friendly talkative woman who knew the Tarbox family inside out. She understood how relentlessly positive, hard-headed and guarded they all were, so when Barb went on about how perfect everything was at home or on her crusade, Little Barb would call her on it, telling her she knew it had to be difficult and messy. Barb appreciated Little Barb's attitude and let down her walls, unloading her own frustrations about her cancer, about Pat, Tracy and everyone else.

Monday, March 3. Dozens and dozens of e-mails and letters of encouragement were coming in to Barb, more than ever before. She showed me her favourite note. "I'm 65 years old and have smoked for 53 years," Gail Parsons of Red Deer wrote. "Your tremendous courage has made you my mentor, and I am in the process of becoming a non-smoker. God bless you. When you get to heaven, please give my love to my dad and twin sister, Gilda, both of whom died of cancer. They are now totally free of pain and enjoying eternal serenity, as you will be."

Patients at the Cross Cancer Institute treated Barb as a conquering hero. They hugged her, thanked her, gave her flowers and cards. She had entered that realm of celebrity where strangers called her by her first name. For her part, Barb always asked questions and offered encouragement.

On her first morning of the new treatment, she marched into the radiology ward, smiling, laughing, chatting up the staff. She was keen to get started, she

---

Opposite page: Barb says goodbye to radiology technician Marilyn Schmidt after her tenth and final radiation treatment at the Cross Cancer Institute.

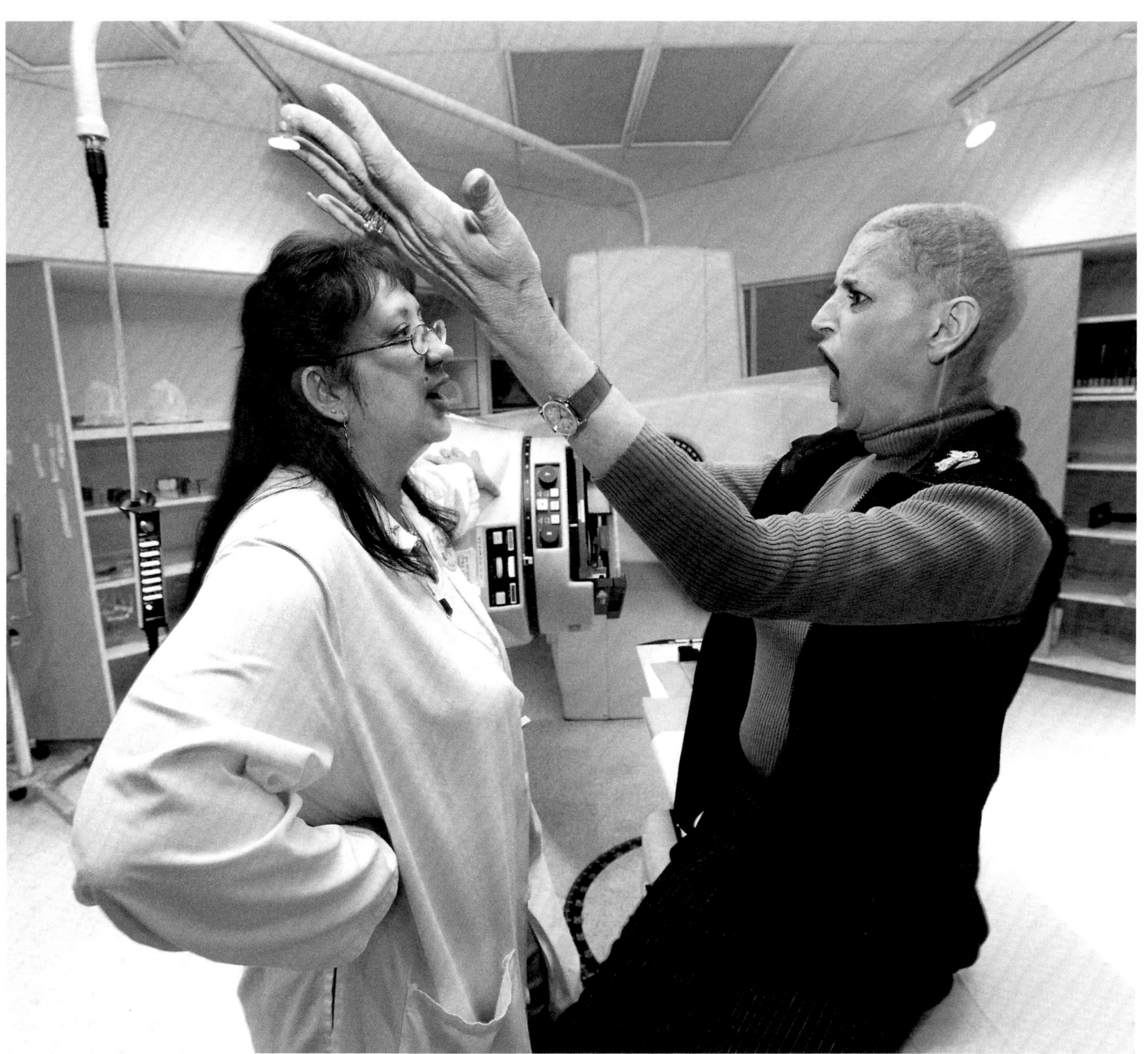

said, even if it meant her hair would fall out again. A fuzz of black, grey and blond curls had grown back in the past few weeks.

"It hasn't made up its mind what colour it's going to be," she said, then laughed. "The next objective is to be a redhead."

Barb offered some sweets to radiology nurse Marilyn Schmidt, a gregarious woman who was to oversee much of her treatment.

"Chocolate Rolo?" Barb said.

"Chocolate?" Schmidt asked.

"Yeah, two times a day."

"It gets rid of that bitchiness."

"Sweetie, I don't know about that. I used to be able to say that worked for me, but not now that I got all these tumours in my head."

In the treatment room, Barb lay flat on a platform bed. She pulled her form-fitting plastic mask, a new one, over her face.

"Did you save the other mask?" Schmidt asked. "You trying for a collection?"

Schmidt clamped the mask to the platform so Barb's head was fastened securely. The platform whined and raised up. Red laser lights crisscrossed Barb's face, the finders of a lethal weapon, targeting the brain tumours. The nurses left her there.

In the safety of an adjacent room, a nurse punched a computer button and the Theratron Elite 80 radiation unit went to work. Old Faithful, the staff called the machine, with its Cobalt 60 to assault the tumours. In a few minutes, it was over.

"I feel sorry in a sense for this cancer," Barb said on the way out. "It doesn't know my attitude."

She'd gone back to calling her tumours Betty Lou, she said, to hell with the Buddy Holly song, and continued to tell them how much she hated them. She was happy that her body was going to be donated to science, so that Betty Lou could be studied for weaknesses. "When the day comes and they're going to cut Betty Lou out of me, I personally hope they squish the crap out of her."

Tuesday, March 4. "My husband hated my smoking, my children hated it and I wasn't willing to stop," April Paris of Calgary wrote to Barb. "Then about two years ago I started coughing at night. Even that didn't make me stop. I have seen all the commercials and it didn't mean anything. And then came you, daughter, model, wife, mother and now educator. I just want to thank you from the bottom of my heart."

Wednesday, March 5. "I must be blunt: you scared the **** out of me," Andrew Shapiro, a student from Lower Canada College in Montreal, e-mailed Barb. "I thought you were going to give us this little speech on how we shouldn't smoke, blah, blah, blah, but you really left an impression. . . Not every single person you spoke to will either quit smoking or never try it. But the one person you affected, me, adds one more to that growing list."

Donna Gingera sent out an e-mail outlining the National Film Board's ambitious plans for filming Barb in a number of settings. In the end, it proved too much for Barb, especially as the radiation therapy sapped her. The project fell through.

At the Cross, I had a long talk with Pat. He'd taken

over Barb's pill intake, he said, and had to give her heck once in a while because Barb would eat certain foods, like chocolate, that didn't sit well with her medications.

"She's always liked the junk food. She likes meat and potatoes."

Pat was glad Barb wasn't speaking at any schools during her current treatment. "Tracy needs a little break, too. Today, Barb is pretty good, and I'm hoping it's the direct result of the radiation maybe starting to shrink it down already. Her speech is better."

When her treatment was done, however, he expected her to get back to the schools. "I just told her, 'When it gets too much to do three schools a week, do two. I'm not telling you to stop, but you have to slow down, because if not, your body will tell you to slow down, and you'll be down to zero.'

"She's adding closure to everything in her life," he continued. "If she has to leave this earth and she knows she's going to save one, ten, a hundred, a thousand people from developing cancer, then she did what she could when she was here. She was productive on this earth. That keeps her going. From what I gather, this is hitting three generations: the kids she's talking to right now, them pestering their parents about not smoking, and them making sure their own kids don't smoke. You can't measure how many people this will go across."

As much as Barb talked about her illness, Pat said he didn't feel the need to talk with his own friends about it. He'd never once brought up her illness with his best friend of 37 years. "He's kind of freaked out about it. That's fine."

I told Pat that Tracy had been mad at him for not taking Barb to more talks. He said he'd never heard that from Tracy. He had offered his help to Barb, he said, but she shut him down, saying, "It's OK. Tracy wants to take me."

After that, Pat said, he just backed off.

He wasn't hurt if Tracy felt resentful towards him, he said. "People's feelings and emotions are so highly charged right now with everything that is happening."

In fact, Pat said he was grateful to Tracy. "To have a friend that is that dedicated and that close and that loving is so important."

What did her friendship mean to Barb?

"The hugs. The friendly shoulder to cry on. I know Barb — as much as my daughter and myself — she doesn't want to break down in front of us, so it's good to have a friend around so you do have a moment where if you lose it, you have somebody who cares about you."

The Tarbox family liked to put up a brave front, Pat said. "We're terrible that way. I can see it in my daughter already. I know Barb went through a little bit with Mackenzie at the beginning. They kind of got it out in the open, doing a lot of hugging and crying and hand holding. Mackenzie had concerns. 'Oh, Dad works all the time, who is going to be around? Am I going to be by myself?' "

Pat said he'd assured Mackenzie that he'd be there, and reminded her that when Barb had worked for a year, he had driven her to school almost every day.

"I don't believe I've let anybody down so far," Pat said. "And I won't. My family knew that, too, that if anything they could always depend on me. And they do."

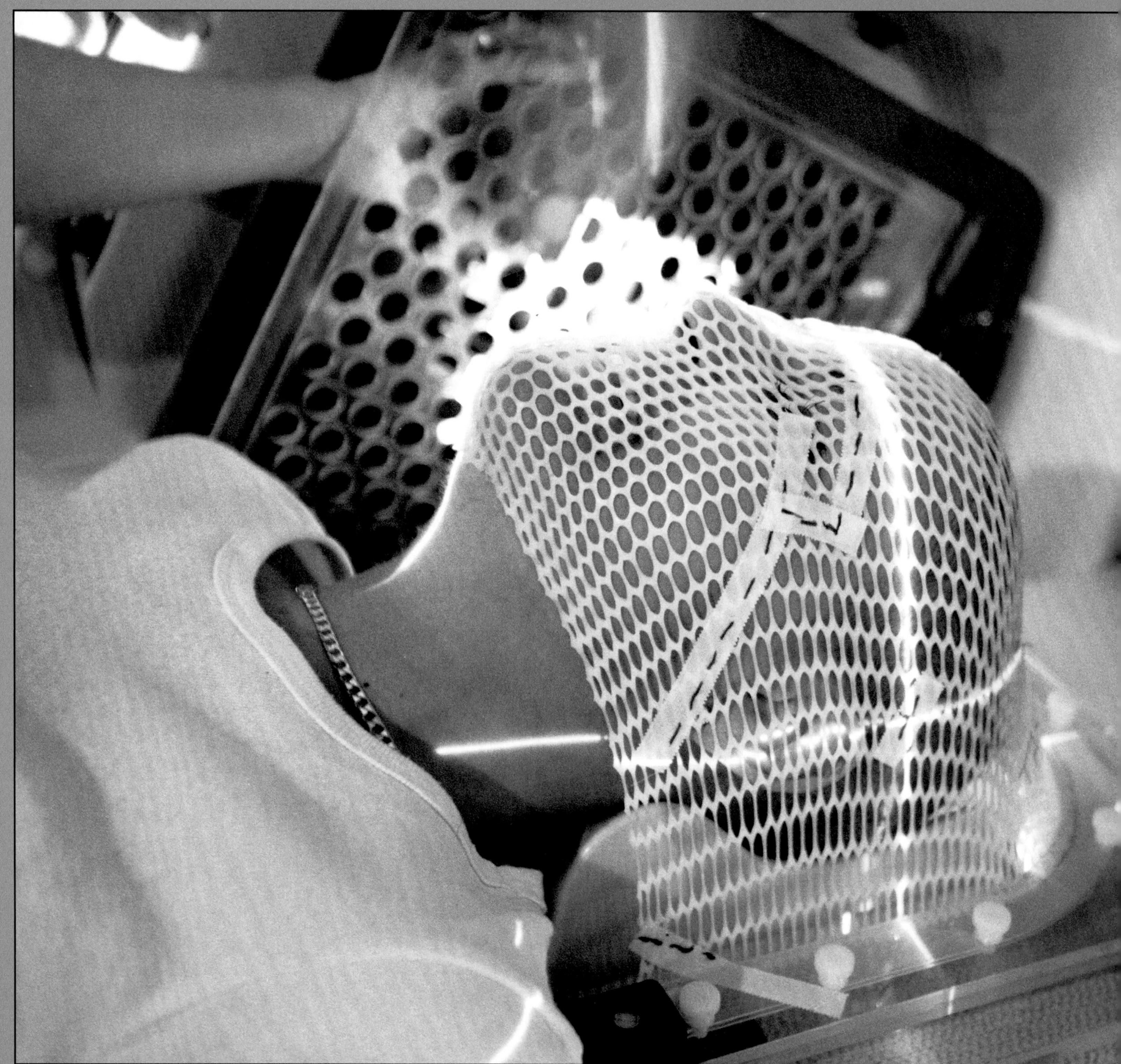

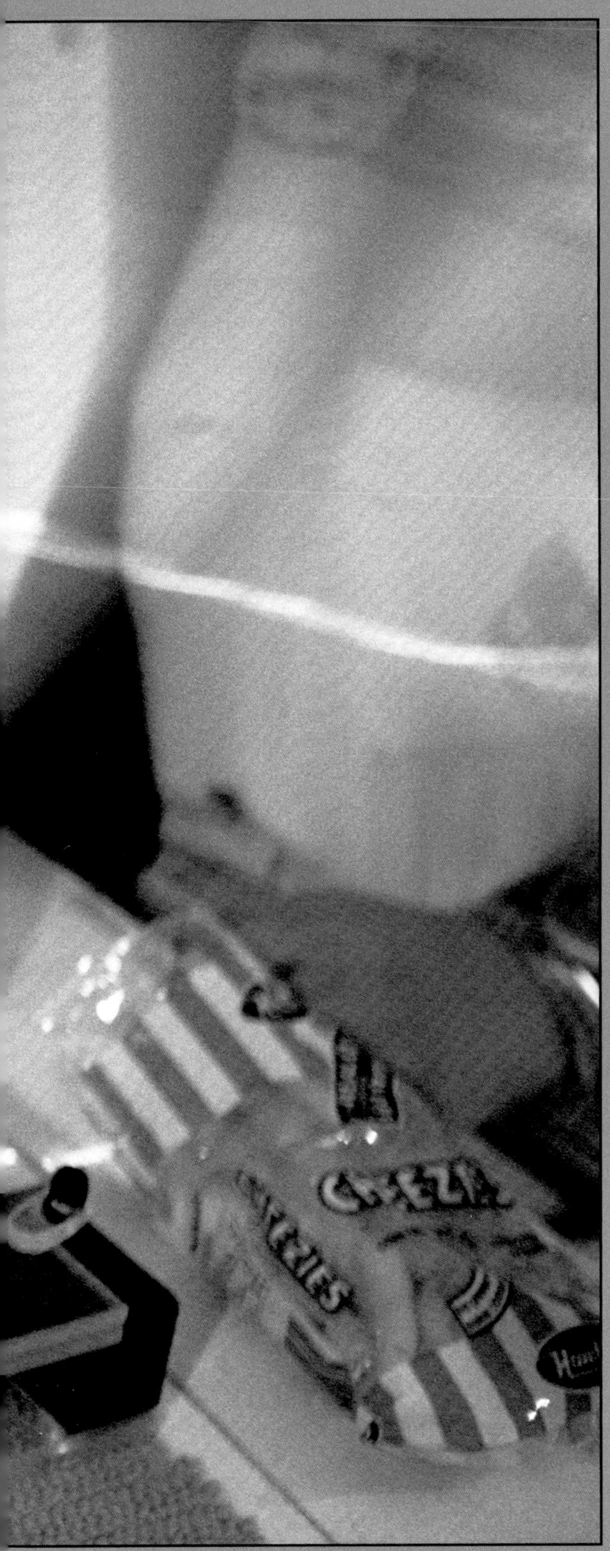

Barb receives radiation. This time, she forgets she has a snack with her and has to leave the Cheezies on the bed behind her head.

Barb's head was fastened securely. The platform whined and raised up. Red laser lights crisscrossed Barb's face, the finders of a lethal weapon, targeting the brain tumours . . . The Theratron Elite 80 radiation unit went to work. Old Faithful, the staff called the machine, with its Cobalt 60 to assault the tumours.

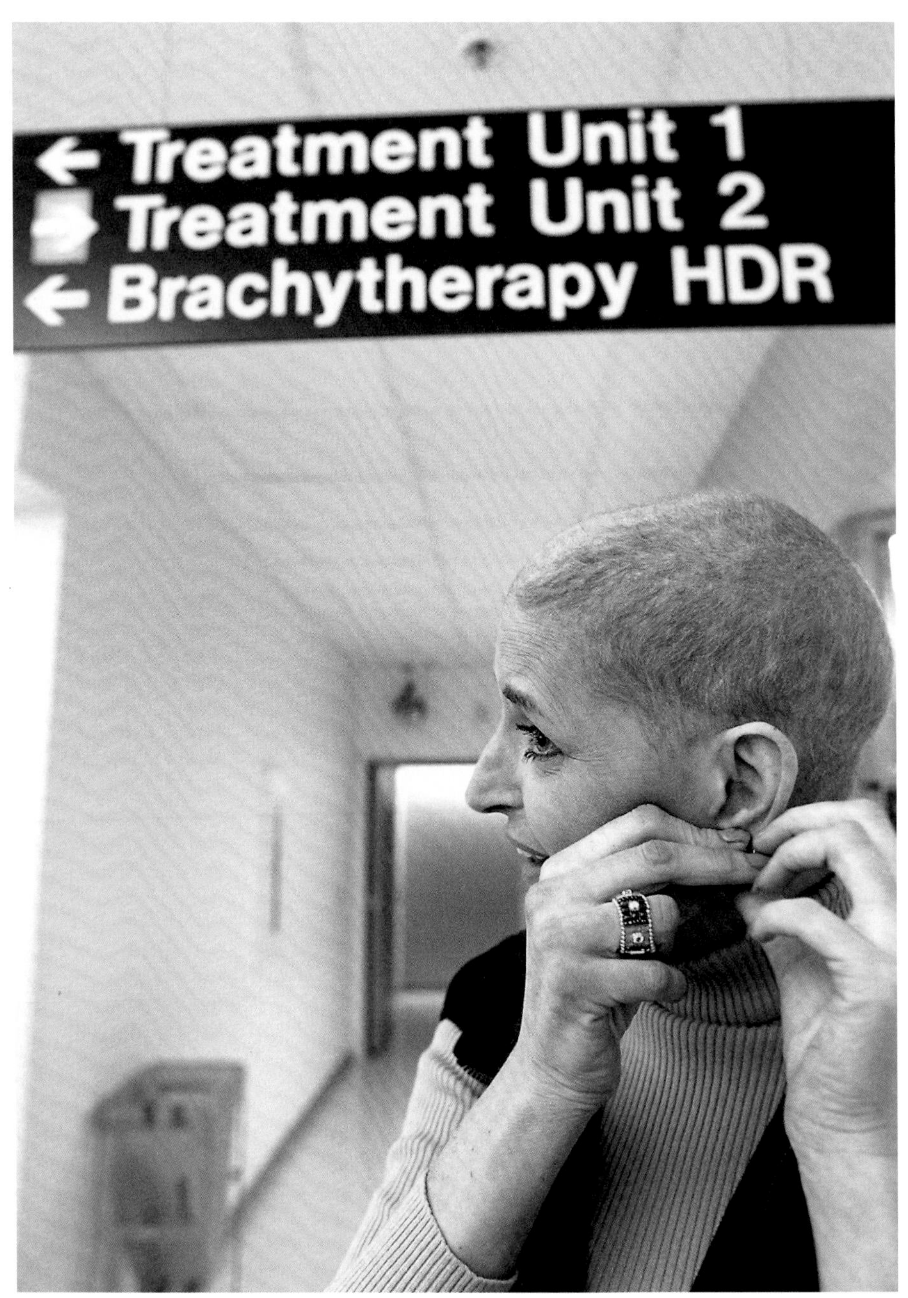

Barb puts her earrings on after receiving radiation.

Thursday, March 6. At the Cross Cancer, a man named Roy Trosin showed up to present Barb with a bouquet of flowers. Trosin told Barb he was the truck driver who had heard her on Al Stafford's CHED radio show just before Christmas and had quit smoking right then. Barb gave him a hug. Pat shook his hand.

That night, Barb appeared on the Stafford show again, her regular monthly visit. One caller told Stafford that he'd just spent $10 on a pack of cigarettes. "I thought if I can talk to Barb, and she tells me to do it, I'll quit."

Barb told him that life is incredible and he never would want to face cancer.

"OK, this is all I needed to hear," the caller said. "When I get home I'm going to throw that ten dollars in the garbage."

Amazing, I thought. People were now treating Barb as if she really were a saint. One touch, one word, and they believe they're healed.

Another caller asked Barb if she had quit smoking. Barb stumbled about in answering, saying smoking made her angry, and that she should never have started, but never clearly admitting she was still doing it, let alone smoking heavily. Stafford pressed her, pointing out that so many people had quit since she started her crusade, so why not her, too?

"What are they going to do?" Barb replied, deflecting the question. "Wait until they're diagnosed, and then not have a chance, where it won't make a difference to quit?"

"But I'm not talking about them, I'm talking about you."

"Will it make a difference with me? No."

"No, of course, but why not quit anyway? Haven't you given the tobacco industry enough?"

"I've given them my life."

Barb sounded hurt now. But Stafford didn't relent: "But you're still spending money on that product. Why?"

"OK, let's get serious, not as much money. I don't have the strength. I sit down and I look at the cigarette and it's a power struggle between the cigarette and me."

On this one question, Barb's gift of gab failed her. Her main problem was her continued embarrassment over her smoking, which kept her from answering questions about the issue directly, and kept her from defending her ongoing habit.

Smoking calmed her, I saw that clearly, and she needed calm during this stressful time. Why not just say that?

She also had far more serious drugs to worry about than nicotine just now, such as morphine and other powerful medications. At this point in her life, living under a death sentence, smoking was a paltry concern. It was no longer an evil for her, even if it remained a great evil for others. But Barb was too flustered by the issue to ever defend herself forcefully.

That night when she got home, several encouraging e-mails awaited her, including one from Rhonda Sargent, who had listened to the CHED show. Sargent had been driving from Red Deer to Edmonton that evening and thanked Barb for a timely intervention. "Today I found myself in a gas station buying a pack of cigarettes and then lighting up one on the highway. Once again, I was totally disappointed in myself. I was at the Ponoka area when I heard you come on the radio. THERE IS A GOD!!! I listened to you for about

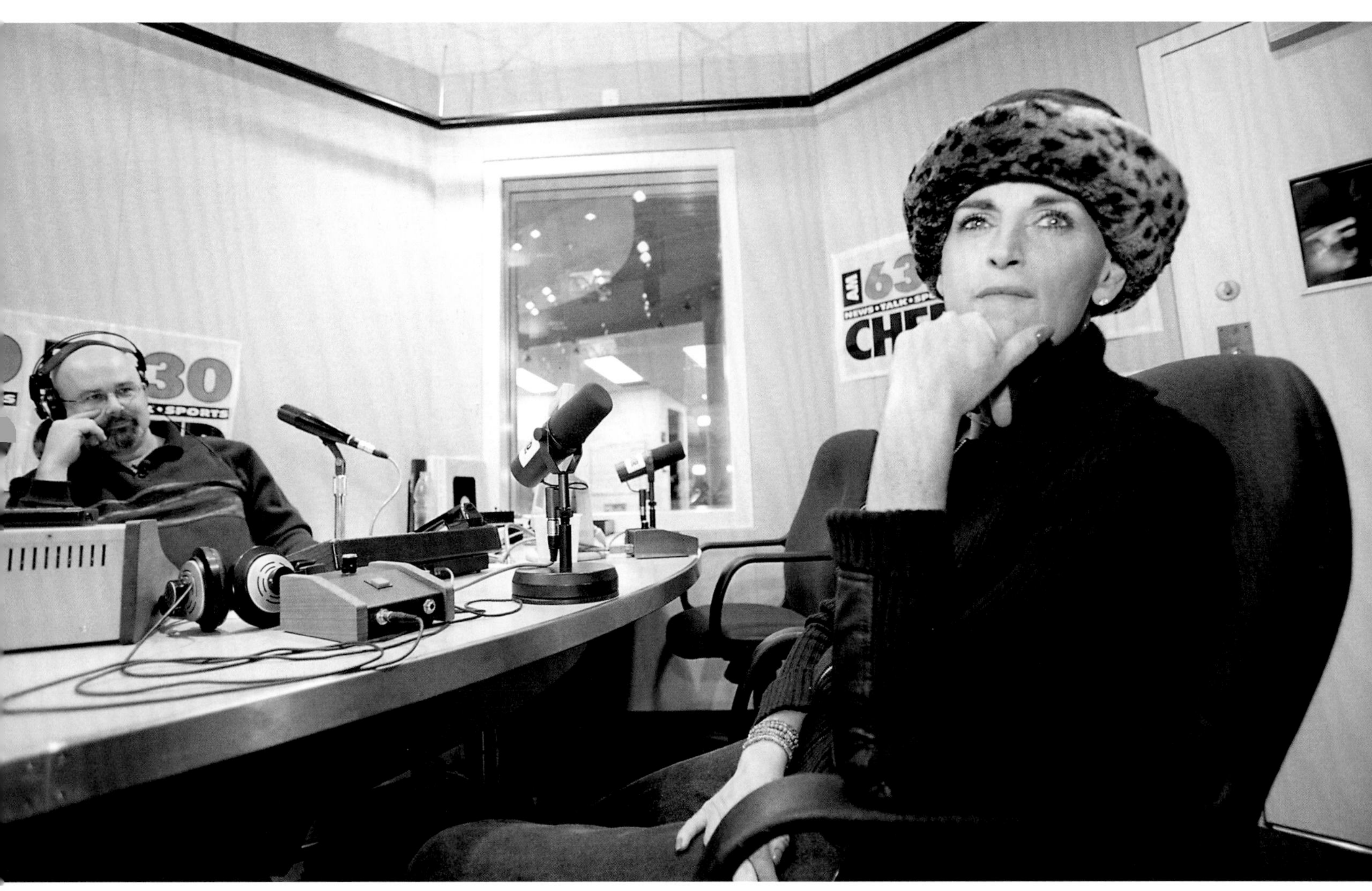

Barb waits for a commercial to end as she does one of many appearances on the Al Stafford show.

twenty minutes and threw them out the window. I will never smoke again."

Friday, March 7. During a visit to the Grey Nuns on February 17, Barb had met a woman with breast cancer, and that woman's daughter, Nicola Verbeek, now sent Barb an e-mail. Her mother had just been through surgery for breast cancer, Verbeek said, and that day there had been complications. "My mother was scared. For the first time in our lives we couldn't just 'make it go away' with a nice bunch of flowers. . . If it hadn't been for the kind words and inspiration you gave her, I don't know if she would have snapped out of it like she has. She has decided that no matter what, she is not going to live her life waiting for cancer to take over. . . I cannot thank you enough."

Saturday, March 8. "I have tried to quit smoking for ten years," Megan Harris, a 37-year-old wife and mother of two from Vancouver e-mailed Barb. "Done the patch, pills and gum!!! I have never been successful. I wanted to write to you to tell you that since December 19th, 2002, after I read your story in the paper, I have never picked up another cigarette again!"

Tracy made a call to book a get-together for her extended family and Barb and Pat at a South Side restaurant. When she told the manager who the booking was for, he scolded her: "I'm just concerned with your lack of consideration to book in a smoking section with Mrs. Tarbox in attendance."

"Number one, buddy, this is none of your business," Tracy fumed. "Number two, Barb still smokes!"

In the end, Barb bowed out. She had collapsed at home on her couch, exhausted from the radiation. Her bone pain, headaches, nausea and fatigue were all more intense in this second round of therapy. Werner said he understood Barb completely. Ten years back, he'd gone through radiation therapy for testicular cancer, and it had left him so wiped, he couldn't think of anything but sleep, he said. It was as if he had a terrible flu all day long.

Sunday, March 9. Little Barb worried it was too hard on Mackenzie to be home alone with Barb in the evening when Pat was at work, but for her part, Mackenzie took pride in her role. She started to help nurse her mom, getting her blankets, or water and pop to drink.

"Mom, if you wouldn't mind, I don't want to go out and play," Mackenzie said to Barb in the morning. "I want to look after you."

"You don't have to look after me," Barb said. "Just stay and cuddle and watch TV."

But Mackenzie needed breaks, too. Throughout Barb's ordeal, she had continued to excel at school. She appeared to relish going, making Pat think that school was a respite for her, just like hockey, darts and his own work were for him. But school wasn't always easy for Mackenzie. One student had teased her cruelly: "Your mommy is dying because she deserves it. She should have quit smoking."

After that, Mackenzie came home seething, not at the girl, but at her mom for her smoking, and for always being so tired and ill. Mackenzie stewed over the issue, but at last told Barb what the girl had said.

Barb told Mackenzie she shouldn't worry about other kids. "Sometimes kids say things they don't think about. They don't realize how it hurts another kid's heart."

It wasn't easy to handle Mackenzie, Barb told me. Part of her wanted to go out shopping and buy Mackenzie everything she'd ever wanted. But Barb refrained from spoiling her, and continued to discipline her as if things were normal, taking her allowance away when she didn't clean her room.

Monday, March 10. For the first time today, Barb talked freely with me about how much she needed her cigarettes, even now. After her radiation session, Tracy, Barb and I had gone out for lunch at the University of Alberta Earl's burger location. Barb picked away at a beef dip sandwich.

I asked about CHED's Al Stafford peppering her with questions about her smoking on his show.

"You do get tired of hearing the same questions," she said, "but they are the right questions. I deserve the criticism. I don't get mad at people. I will kick my butt until the final day. I am the best example of an addiction ever. "

I'd heard Barb attack her habit many times, but I put it to her that, in fact, she still loved to smoke.

"It's like you're adrenalized by the need," she admitted. "I can feel it rising. I can feel agitation. You can feel it. I start to anticipate. It's an incredible feeling — *I have to have that cigarette*! I need that first drag in the morning. It has to be, or the day will not start."

At last, the truth.

Tracy had just told me the story about Barb's discovery of asparagus back in February.

Was she still eating the stuff?

Barb screwed up her face, as if she'd tasted a horrible food. "Can I just say I do not like asparagus?" she said and laughed. "I'm meat and potatoes. I always have been. I had three bites and said, 'At least I can say I tried it.' It's just not for me."

She had had it with miracle cures, she said, but pitches from homeopaths and faith healers were still flooding in. "I get offended when others say they have a cure. Some companies are just outright outrageous. They show no respect for our medical community. If we had a cure for cancer, the medical community would know about it. That's why I don't worry about it."

She admired her doctors, she said, and had made up her mind not to be like so many patients who got angry at the medical staff, taking out their suffering on them.

I told Barb she'd been doing very well in that regard in recent weeks.

She shook her head. "Don't make me out to be a hero because I'm far from it."

Barb and Tracy were getting along well again, I noticed, Tracy not too stressed, Barb calmer, relaxed, quick to laugh.

It was a fascinating time for her, she said, meeting all these people, all of them on such different paths. The possibilities for people seemed endless, she said. What would they do with their lives? Where would they go?

She was just glad to be around to ask those questions, she said.

"I feel more grateful now for the small things, for the smell of fresh snow on the trees. Feeling cold is OK. That I can still feel it is great. Now I am walking and I see the line-ups in stores and it's OK. I can wait. Seeing the faces of the kids and you look in the eyes of people, the sparkles! People are incredible. My car gets dirty and that didn't used to please me, but now it does. There's a lot to be grateful for."

She returned to my original question, about Stafford asking about her smoking. "I look at it this way, that God gave me the gift of gab, and for that I'm grateful. I just say what I feel, some people like it, sometimes they don't. They're fed up with my smoking. But I'm not offended."

Wednesday, March 12. Rosa Bidner of Ottawa sent Barb a note, thanking her for getting her 17-year-old daughter at Hillcrest high school to quit. "My constant nagging and warning her that smoking could kill went unheard. She was becoming a seasoned smoker. When she got up in the morning, it would be the first thing she did. Have a cigarette. When I would pick her up from school, the strong smell of smoke would fill the car and fill my heart with fear that my daughter would end up with cancer at a young age. Your message has changed all that."

It was the eighth day of radiation, and Barb had had enough of smelling herself burning. "You always get that god awful smell. The first time I smelled it, it was, 'Gee, did someone not clean up?'"

Barb had a checklist of the symptoms that people experience just before death. When she went down it, she saw she had most of them. "My body is ready now. The weakness in it is phenomenal. When I'm having trouble pulling myself up four steps with both hands, that is a problem."

Mackenzie had told her that she would always be right there and catch her if she fell. Barb told me she loved her daughter's intent, but had chuckled to herself when Mackenzie said this, thinking, *that'd be quite the catch for a little girl.*

Thursday, March 13. Barb brought in Cheezies to the Cross, handed the bag to Marilyn Schmidt. "You got to eat," Barb said.

"Yeah, I'm dwindling away to nothing," Schmidt laughed.

Barb lay down on the treatment table, ready to have her head immobilized.

Pat was now spending more time at home, she told Schmidt. "I tell him, 'Isn't there something else you could do? Go play hockey!'"

She said she liked it when Pat was at the rink so she could listen to loud country music. Schmidt nodded. "Guys in tight jeans, that's what it's all about."

"You got it, sweetie," Barb said.

At the end of the session, Marilyn handed back the bag of Cheezies to Barb. "Take them."

"Why?"

"Because you need the weight more than I do. Your thighs are smaller than my arms."

Tracy, Barb, Greg and I all went out for lunch. Barb had seven sugars in her coffee. Tracy said she'd put just four in one day, and Barb had gagged on it. Not sweet enough.

Barb had a bandage on her finger. She was sitting on the couch, she explained, watching TV and smoking, when she had fallen asleep. The cigarette had burnt right down, frying two fingers. She was now worried about burning her house down. Her new rule, she said, was when she wasn't smoking, she would put the cigarette in an ashtray.

Barb left the table to go the washroom.

"Barb is different," Tracy said just then. "She's way different. She's back to being the way she was before. She is happy and smiling."

I agreed whole-heartedly. I relished my time with her now, and found myself admiring her in a new way, not for her dynamism in front of a crowd, but for her way with Greg and Tracy, and with nurses, clerks, strangers. As sick as she was, she would stop, smile, ask questions, laugh, hand out a compliment. She had a remarkable ability to find the right words to put others at ease.

This mental image of Barb was influencing my own behaviour, I realized.

I was always busy, doing my work with Barb, writing other feature stories, as well as a weekly column. At home, I was the father of three sons, with shared custody of them, meaning I cared for them at my house three-to-four days out of every week. I was also newly married and loved to be with my wife. To meet my responsibilities and do all I wanted, I had to move fast. That wasn't about to change.

But now, when I walked by the security guard at my office, I found myself stopping, saying hello, finding out his name, chatting a bit.

When I talked to my bosses, I relaxed, let down my guard, asked about their lives, said more about my own.

When I was with my boys, I didn't just think about getting them supper, getting them to school, working with them on homework. Sometimes, I looked for that sparkle in their eyes.

All these things I'd seen in Barb.

In Tracy's mind, Barb was back to being her old self, but I thought I saw something more. Barb was in a new place, it seemed to me. She saw the world through new eyes and it was a world transfigured. I had expected her to become more distant as she got closer to death. Instead, she was pulling ever more closely to others. It was as if she saw her beloved Michael in all of us now, not just in Luc Caouette, but in everyone and everything she met. She wanted to love and hold and nurture all her friends, all the nurses, all the people in the check-out lines. She cherished each moment, even the cold days, the descending snow, the grime on her car.

Friday, March 14. Edmonton's long-time anti-smoking advocate Les Hagen, director of Action on Smoking and Health (ASH), had contacted Barb and asked her to lend her support to a proposed provincial government bill that would ban smoking in all public places. The Tarbox Bill, it would be called, Hagen said. Barb was all for it, and was determined to meet with Alberta's Premier Ralph Klein.

"Klein won't be able to say, 'No,' to me," she told Marilyn Schmidt at the Cross.

"I know."

"He doesn't know what's coming, baby!"

As Barb was leaving, for good this time, the nurses all came out and hugged her.

"It was great meeting you," said radiologist Mike Babchuk.

"You know," Barb said, "I've never had a really exciting life. So this place is exciting."

"Barb," asked another nurse. "Do you want your shell?"

"Yes, please!" Barb took hold of her new plastic mask. "My other one is so dirty."

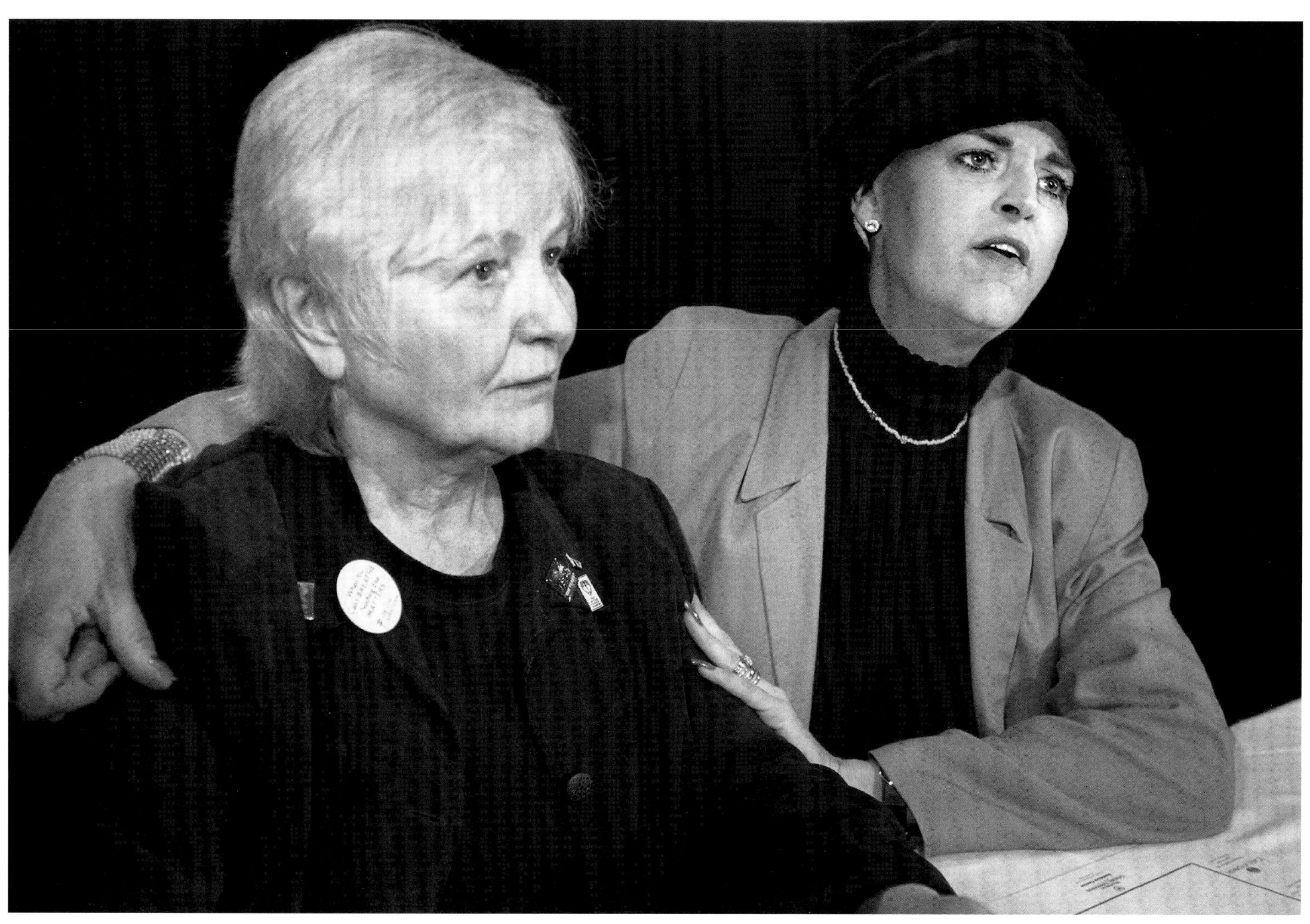

Barb shares the stage with anti-smoking crusader Heather Crowe during a luncheon meeting.

Saturday, March 15. Chris Maksylewicz of Edmonton wrote to say his girlfriend Tanya had quit because of Barb. "I pray that Tanya keeps it up, but I didn't think she would. Well, she went to the Sidetrack Café yesterday and got offered just a drag! And she said, 'No.' YEAH!!!! She also thought of you and said a little prayer."

Monday, March 17. Edmonton city council was amending its anti-smoking bylaw, with anti-smoking councillors hoping to push through a ban on smoking in bars, nightclubs, casinos and bingos.

Barb agreed to speak at a public hearing at City Hall. She was scheduled to talk first thing in the morning. As we waited for proceedings to start, I talked to Tracy, who was in a fine mood. She said she'd gone out shopping on her own for three hours on Sunday, the first time she'd done that in six months. She bought a sharp blue blazer, and had it on today.

The chairperson called Barb to the microphone.

"I'm asking you to prohibit smoking in all public places," Barb said. "Anyone on earth can walk into a restaurant, sit down for one hour and not have to light up, even me. Six months ago, I may not have said that, but one day go down to the Cross Cancer Institute. You'll soon change your mind."

To rally public opinion, the Alberta Lung Association brought in another dynamo of the anti-smoking movement, Heather Crowe of Ottawa.

Crowe was 57 years old, but had never smoked. Instead, she worked for 40 years as a waitress in restaurants where the air was often blue with smoke. That smoke had triggered tumours in her lung and lymph node. Her doctor told her she had a 15-per-cent chance of being alive in five years.

Crowe billed herself as the "canary in the coal mine" of the hospitality industry. Second-hand smoke kills as many as 7,800 Canadians each year, through heart disease, lung cancer, respiratory disease and other ailments, anti-smoking advocates say. Yet two-thirds of Canadians still work in environments where smoking is allowed.

Barb wanted to meet Crowe, so after giving her speech, she headed over to Crowe's news conference at the nearby Sheraton Hotel. Barb sat and watched as reporters questioned Crowe, a soft-spoken and serious-minded woman. She then joined Crowe at the head table. The two women hugged. They couldn't be more different: Barb the smoker, tall and talkative, flamboyant in her black leather skirt and electric blue blouse; Heather the non-smoker, short and quiet, a bit rumpled, cords, brown jacket, black blouse.

Barb's advanced illness shocked Crowe. She dreaded her fate all the more. At the press conference, though, she contained any fears.

"Oh I admire you so much," Barb told her. "And you know what? We're not going to stop, sweetie, until our message comes through. If anybody ever turns around to you and says, 'This will never, ever happen,' look at us."

"Take a look," Crowe said. "We know. We're not going to be here much longer. Smoking kills."

"At 41, my life is over."

"57, finished."

"All because I took a drag."

"And I had to earn a living. I went to

Newfoundland and the girls working in the bars were all on antihistamines. And there was one waitress in her 50s and she had holes drilled in her sinuses just to keep her job."

Looking on, Les Hagen, director of ASH, smiled widely. He said seeing Crowe and Barb together was the most powerful thing he'd experienced in his 15 years as an anti-smoking advocate. "It's uncanny that two national champions of tobacco control come together at the same time with the same message. They're having more impact on raising the profile of this issue than all the health organizations combined."

Afterwards, I talked with Crowe, who told me she wasn't mad at the smokers at her old restaurants, that many of them didn't know better. "I'm not asking them to give up a natural bodily function, just to step outside to smoke, and to let us have our health."

She had little sympathy for restaurant and nightclub owners who said anti-smoking bylaws hurt their business. "As a worker in that kind of environment, it was like a gas chamber and you're sending others in there to perish. I don't know where the owner thinks that he has the right to sacrifice these workers."

Tuesday, March 18. Barb had hoped that after her radiation therapy ended, she would feel renewed vigour. Instead, she felt like she was falling apart. If she brushed by the couch, her leg would bruise. Her skin flaked and blistered. She shuffled when she walked, moving like someone ancient.

CFRN had scheduled an interview with Barb at Tracy's house. When Barb tried to climb the steps there, she collapsed. She lay at the door for several minutes, before at last summoning the strength to get up and open it. When she did, she came crashing through, bellowing at Tracy, "Don't let me go anywhere without my cane!"

Wednesday, March 19. "I am just like an alcoholic who loves their liquor," Marnie Molnar of Calgary, a 47-year-old woman with two teenaged daughters, wrote to Barb. "I LOVED smoking. I know this because 17 years ago, I did stop for six months, and all it took was one puff, one night, and I was right back to 20 cigarettes the very next day. . . When I saw your commercial, I cried with you. What kept sinking in until I could bear it no more was, 'I have devastated my husband of 20 years,' and 'I don't want to say good-bye to my daughter.' I tend to be a giver, so I was devastated to think how selfish I have been. . . I made a promise with my girlfriend that when we went on our vacation we would both stop smoking. No habits to remind us, no stress excuses, and Palm Springs is not smoker-friendly. In two days, I am proud to say we will not have had a cigarette for one month."

Like so many in the hospitality industry, Pat wasn't keen about Barb's political stand against smoking. "It's typical of her Irish charm to charge into something without thinking about it," he told me.

While Pat was a non-smoker, he was also a businessman, who strongly favoured allowing smoking at bars. A petition was now circulating at his pub against amending the city's smoking bylaw.

At last, he talked to Barb about his concerns. He didn't want to see her push things the so-called Tarbox Bill, he said, not with the city or the province. A press conference with Les Hagen was planned for the coming week and Pat preferred that Barb not attend it.

"If you really want this bill, go for it, but you're walking on thin ice," he told her. "This crusade of yours is not about politics. This is about you and the kids. Stay out of the political arena as much as they try to drag you in. The rocket has shot you to the moon. Maybe it's time to come back down to earth. Get back to the focus of talking to these kids."

Barb also talked over her political work with Tracy, who said she agreed with Pat, and that there was a big difference between a lady who speaks to kids and a woman who screams at the Premier.

"Why are you fighting everyone else's battles?" Tracy asked.

Barb decided to pull back. She told me she'd always respected Pat's opinions and that's why they'd been together for 20 years. She hadn't known that his pub had started a petition. "I hope the bylaw goes through, but you know what? I have a purpose and that's to talk to the kids, and that's what I'm doing, and that's all."

Friday, March 21. Back in January, Barb had been named the Global Woman of Vision, a monthly honour sponsored by the local TV affiliate. Today, the annual banquet was to be held at a posh downtown hotel to honour all of the monthly winners, including Barb.

Barb, Tracy, Pat, Greg and I attended the luncheon, where announcements were to be made of a Mackenzie Tarbox Education Fund and the Barb Tarbox Legacy Fund, which would distribute money to charities selected by Barb. Both had been pushed for by a local businessman, Mohammed Moussa, owner of La Z Boy Furniture Galleries. He had become Barb's friend and had pledged $25,000 himself over five years to the two funds.

Barb looked sharp in a light purple outfit and black hat. She told me she'd been sleeping all week, but was glad to be out today, and to have the chance to speak, even if she'd been told she could only have two minutes at the mic.

The other honoured guests took their turns speaking. When one of the women went on at length, Barb whispered to me, "That was more than two minutes."

That is *so* Barb, I thought, hungry for the spotlight, hungry for more time, more minutes at the microphone today, more days and weeks later.

She spoke as well and dramatically as ever. When she was done, she looked out at the admiring crowd. "Do you know, you all have a particular sparkle?"

The crowd stood and cheered. Mohammed Moussa then took the stage to announce the two Tarbox funds. He had a smile and twinkling eyes, and seemed to me a short, bald and rotund version of Barb.

"I was touched by Barb, I'll never forget her," he said, then looked around for Barb, who was standing right behind him. "Where is she?"

"I'm hiding. All six feet of me."

Moussa turned and smiled. "I'm deeply in love with this woman."

"It's the hair," Barb said.

Just then, she noticed a photograph of her and Mohammed had been projected on the screen. "I love this picture!" she exclaimed, then turned to Moussa. "You always have great hair days."

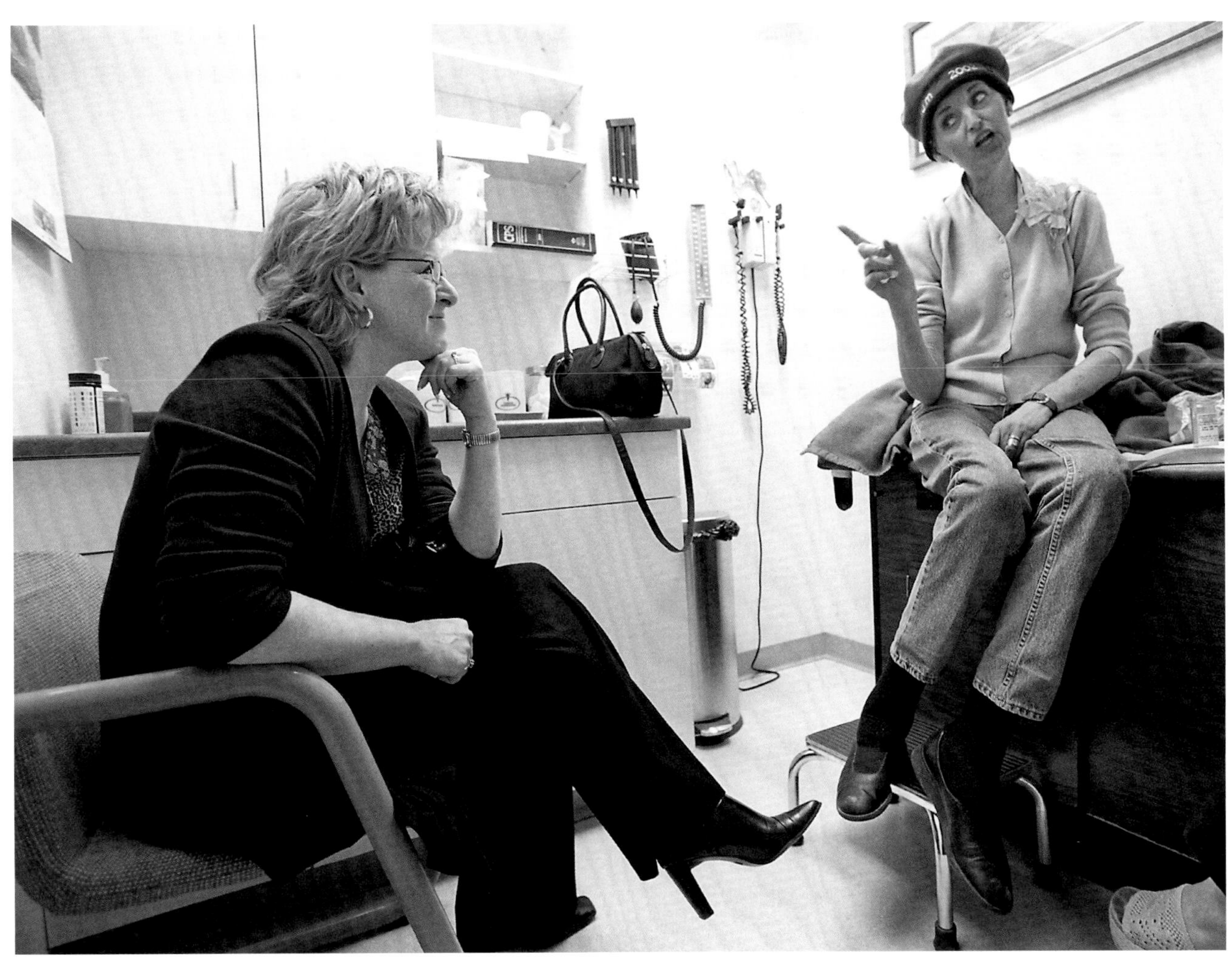

Barb and Tracy, back on the best of terms, talk in Dr. Fonteyne's office.

Sunday, March 23. The sun shone bright and warm. Snow melted in streams along the curb. The weather got Barb thinking about spring cleaning. She wanted to get her winter coat out of her car so she could pack it away for summer. To get to the car, Barb had to climb over a slushy, icy snowbank, the remains of the winter's snow piled along the curb.

Mackenzie offered to help. Barb took her little hand and made it to the top of the bank, but then felt her legs go out from under her. She collapsed to her hands and knees into a puddle of water, rock and mud on the pavement. Her jeans soaked through. Pain rocketed up from her gashed knees.

"Figures! Figures! This is what happens!"
She tried to get up, but her legs wouldn't move.
Tell them to stand up! She instructed herself. *Tell them to stand up!*

"Mommy, I'll help you," Mackenzie said.

Barb looked up to see her daughter wide-eyed with fear.

"You know what, sweetie, if you put your arm underneath my arm, that would help a lot."

Mother and daughter strained. Still Barb didn't move. Minutes passed.

OK, Barb told herself. *Don't freak. Stay calm. Do it for Mackenzie.*

"Oh, look!" Barb said, trying to make a joke. "Now that I'm down here, I might as well be useful. I'll just check out this dirt and make sure the city uses clean dirt on the roads."

Cars whizzed by. Drivers looked over, but no one stopped. Barb felt both resentment and embarrassment.

"Can I call someone?" Mackenzie asked.

"Just give me a few more minutes."

Barb tried to massage her legs. Gradually, feeling came back. At last, she was strong enough that she could pull herself up with Mackenzie's help.

Barb was amazed at how strong her daughter was. When they got inside, Mackenzie went into nurse mode: "Mommy, do you need anything? Can I get you something to drink? Do you need a painkiller? Are you going to phone your nurse?"

"Not yet, sweetie."

"Mommy, aren't you cold?"

"I'm OK, sweetie."

Barb got changed and lay down on the couch, then turned on the electric blanket that Pat had bought for her. After a long time, it warmed her up.

Monday, March 24. The Delta Inn had become our favourite spot for lunch, as it had a comfortable lounge for smoking and a big fire to keep Barb warm. Today, Greg, Tracy and I met with Barb. She ordered a steak sandwich and a salad. She had a good appetite, eating a large portion of her food. She also had five sugars in her coffee. Tracy told me about some of the looks she'd been getting at Tim Horton's when she ordered a small coffee with eight sugars.

Sorry ma'am, the cashier would ask, was that eight sugars?

Yes, Tracy would say.

In the small?

Yes.

When we met now, we would talk about Barb's latest symptoms as always, but spent most of our time chatting about other matters, normal things — family, movies, TV, politics. Barb appreciated it. "I'm so tired of talking about the c-word," she said.

Tracy was still fuming about Barb's terrible fall on the weekend, and how many people had driven by, but no one had stopped.

"That pisses me off. I don't care if it's a kid who has fallen or an adult, you've got to stop."

"I was flippin' furious," Barb said. "I'm not mad now."

"I just about started to cry," Tracy said. "That was so sad."

Over the sound system, B.B. King played. Barb asked a number of questions about the music. She didn't know anything about the blues, she said. Still, she was determined to go out and get her first album.

Again, I admired Barb. At the end of her life, she still hungered for life.

Tuesday, March 25. By a 9-2 vote, Edmonton city council banned smoking in all workplaces and public establishments effective July 1, 2005.

Wednesday, March 26. Barb had been too sick to travel to New York for the Montel Williams show, so a producer and cameraman from the show were hired to interview Pat, Tracy, Barb, Greg and me at the Delta. I was calm for most of the interview, but when the producer asked me about Barb saying good-bye to Mackenzie, I thought about the girl's fate and about my own boys, and had to fight back tears. I was surprised by the intensity of my reaction. I often told myself that I was doing well, that Barb's condition wasn't getting me down. My tears were a reality check.

"I got choked up at that question, also," Tracy later e-mailed me. "I guess we are all human. I told them I don't know how I'm going to say good-bye. I guess it will come from the heart. Barb and I talk all the time and she knows that I love her."

Thursday, March 27. Barb told Dr. Fonteyne that after two hours of being awake, she felt like crashing again. "I have no power in my legs whatsoever. Nausea is the worst. And the weakness. I'm going home to bed. I'm exhausted."

Fonteyne found she had low blood pressure, which could be a result of dehydration. He decided to put her on intravenous at home for her fluids. He would send a homecare nurse to set her up, he said. "You're really dry so I think you'll pep up with more fluid."

"I've never felt this bad before."

"I want you to lay low. I don't want you out and around."

"I am. I'm not doing anything until this is cleared up."

Friday, March 28. In the morning, Tracy e-mailed me to say she'd been over to Barb's the previous night and things had been bad. "She has an I.V. in her chest to help drain the fluid (in her lungs) if need be and to give her the liquids she needs. She is still feeling exhausted this morning, but is very positive and says by Sunday, after fluid intake and meds, she will be raring to go. I love her attitude. She never ceases to amaze me."

Monday, March 31. "Barb is still very dehydrated," Tracy e-mailed me in the late afternoon. "She said she is down to half a pack of smokes a day, which she said is not a good sign. That's what happens at the end, she said."

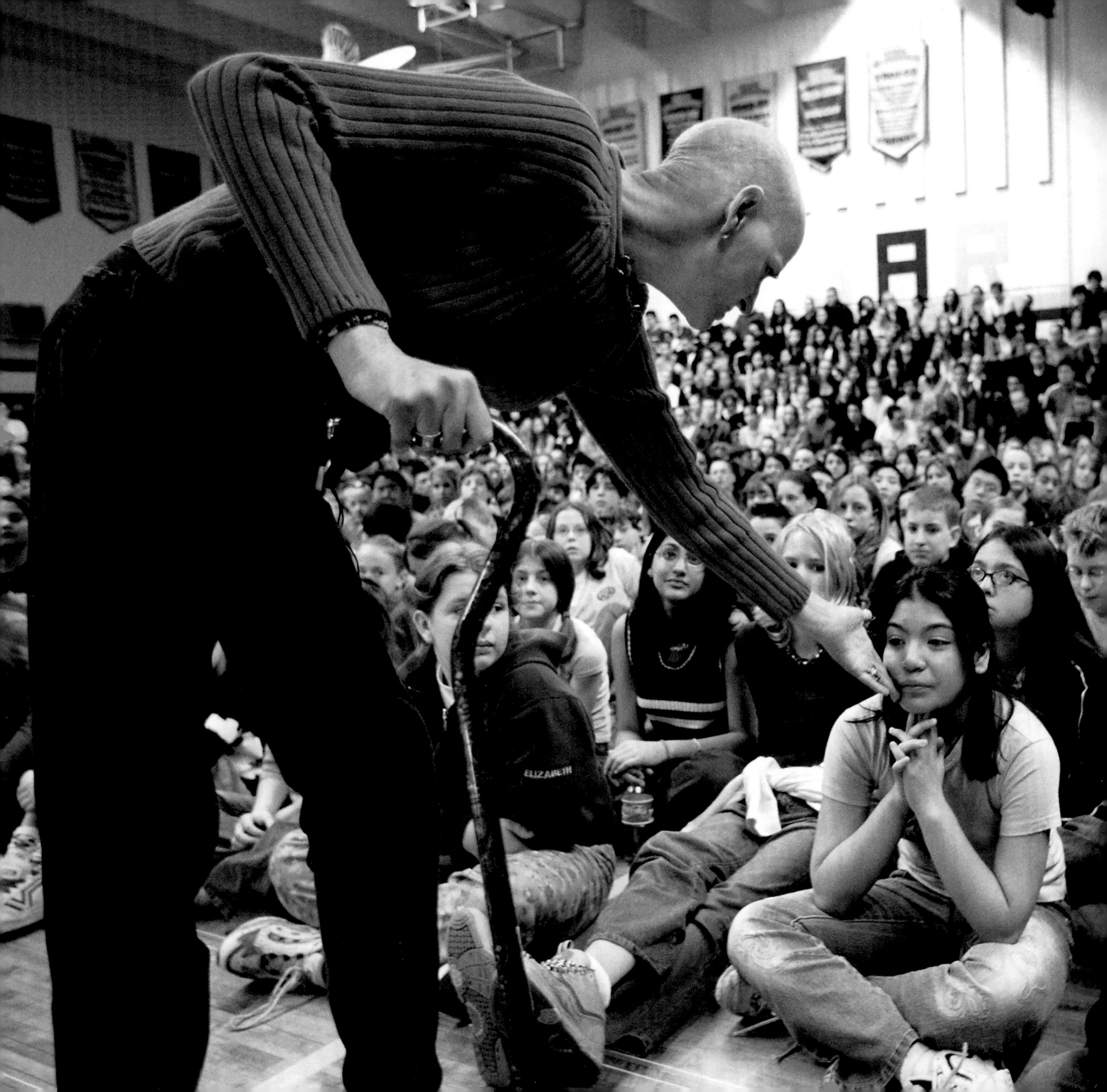
ELIZABETH

April
2 0 0 3

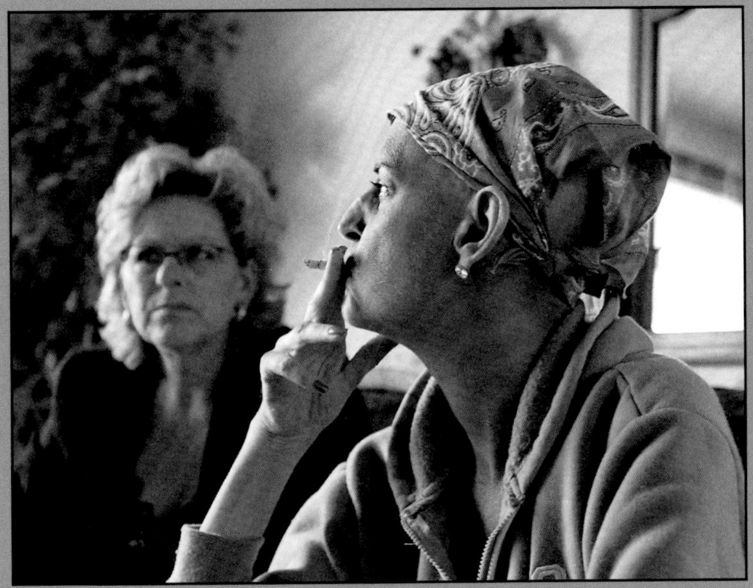

I am ill because of wounds to the soul, to the deep emotional self
and the wounds to the soul take a long, long time, only time can help
and patience, and a certain difficult repentance,
long, difficult repentance, realisation of life's mistake . . .

D. H. Lawrence

Tuesday, April 1. Tracy and the rest of us had previously worried Barb was doing too many public talks. Now we feared she would never do another. She had gone five weeks without speaking at a school. She talked about going, but when Tracy suggested she book a school, Barb invariably would say they should wait until next week, that maybe she would feel better by then.

Did she just want to do one more presentation, a big one, go out with a bang, Tracy finally asked.

"Could you do that?" Barb replied. "I might be going there in a wheelchair, but I want to do it."

Thursday, April 3. I met Barb and Tracy in the foyer of the Edmonton's old Hudson Bay building, now offices of the A-Channel and its *Big Breakfast* TV show, where Barb had been invited to appear. She went partly because some time ago she'd had a dream about the hosts of the show, Steve Antle and Mark Scholz. They were all dancing in the dream, Barb said.

"What kind of dancing?" I asked.

"A different kind of dancing," Barb said and blushed. "I'm not going into it any more."

We all laughed.

Barb had her I.V. tube taped to her shirt. The injection port went into her back. The nurses had first attempted to place the injection site in her arm, Barb said, but that hadn't worked. Her arm had swelled up three times its normal size.

We sat waiting on tall bar stools at a guest coffee counter. A new outlet of the *Winners* discount chain was opening downtown that day, Barb said, and she'd been invited to come in for a special shopping spree half an hour before the main doors opened. "That will stay with you for life!" she said of the spree. "My God, can you imagine!"

"What would you get?" Tracy asked.

"Whatever looks nice."

On camera, we heard host Mark Scholz saying, "I'm getting ready to talk to Barb Tarbox. If you haven't heard her name, you've been living on a different planet."

In her interview, Barb told Scholz her new goal was to speak to 100,000 kids, if only she had the energy. "It's a miracle I'm still steady. It's a miracle."

Sunday, April 6. A new setback hit the Tarbox family; Pat suffered a collapsed lung after he hit a rut in the ice and crashed into the boards during a late-night pick-up hockey game. He needed an emergency operation to drain the lung and was hospitalized at the Royal Alexandra hospital.

It looked like Pat would be in the hospital for a few days at least, Barb told me. She wasn't doing well, either. Her naps weren't naps anymore, but were full-blown sleeps, five or six hours long. To get her in and out of her car, Tracy had to lift her legs.

Her doctor had told Barb she was supposed to take a sip of water every few minutes. Tracy thought Barb was drinking too much pop, which didn't help with her dehydration problem. She told Barb to try ice chips.

"She's going to die of starvation," Tracy told me later in the afternoon. "You've got to get something in

---

Opposite page: Barb visits Pat in the Royal Alexandra hospital after Pat suffered a collapsed lung while playing hockey.

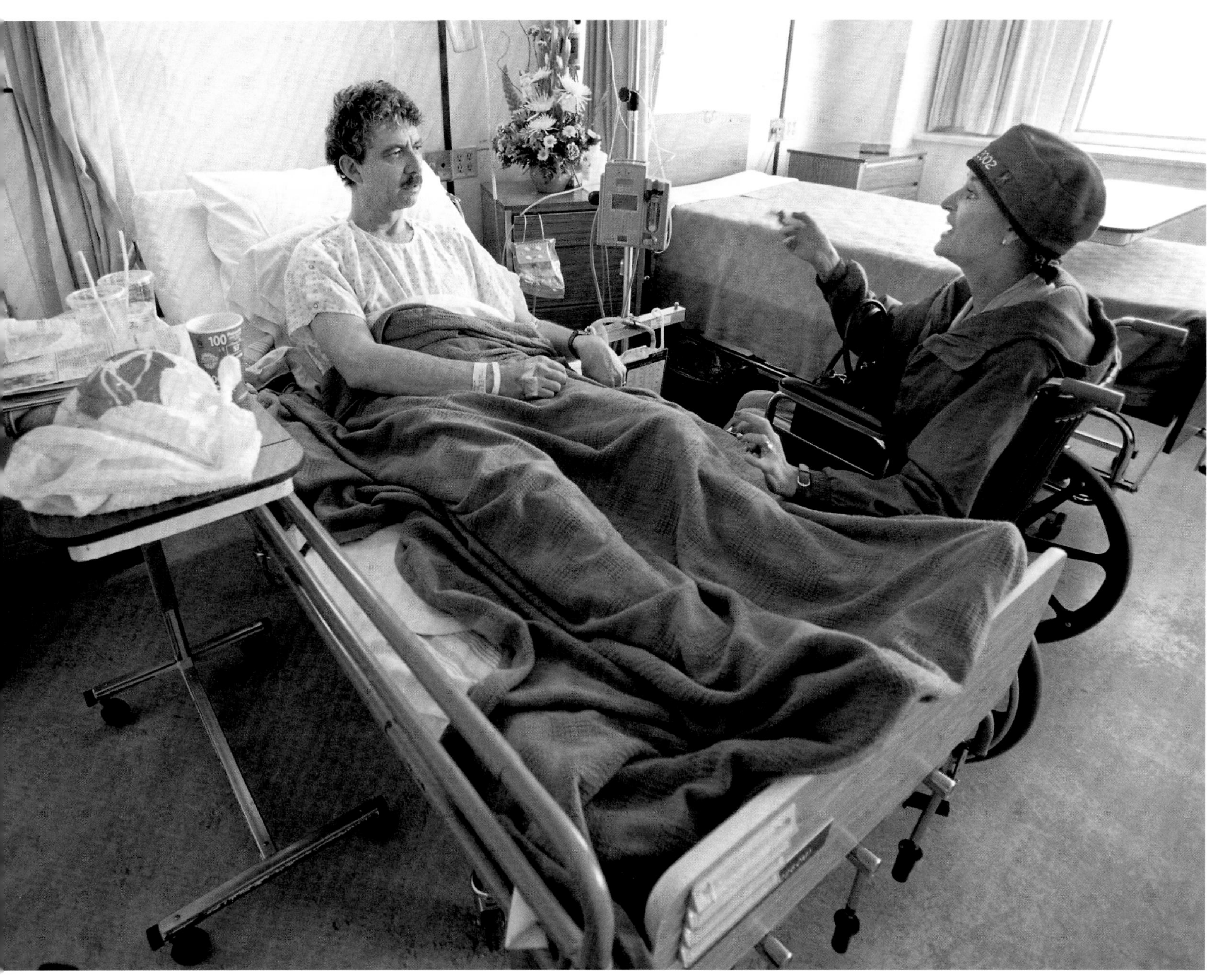
100

you besides this caffeine shit. But how can you deny her something she wants? And she wants caffeine and Coke."

Monday, April 7. Tracy couldn't get hold of Barb all weekend. She left messages, but Barb was too tired to do anything, even return phone calls.

Tuesday, April 8. Barb walked into the lounge at the Delta Inn and asked the waitress to turn on the fireplace.

"I'm frozen," she said.

It was good to see her moving. She appeared as full of energy as ever. So long as she dearly wanted to do something, she was still able to get up off that couch.

She ordered the chicken salad. "My goal is to gain 60 pounds," she said. "I don't think I'm asking for too much."

In her coffee, however, she had only two sugars. "I don't know. I just don't like the sweet taste any more."

"Which is good," Tracy said, "because you don't want sugar dehydrating you."

She took a few bites of her chicken salad and was pleased with that. "Today, I'm going to force myself to have toasted white bread with maple syrup."

Her 42nd birthday was coming up on Thursday. A large party was planned for her favourite eatery, Grub Med. As Tracy helped Barb into her van for the ride home, Barb turned to Greg and me. "I'm going to hook up some of Yiannis's special coffee in an I.V. bottle," she said and laughed. "Think of it this way: it's probably the last time."

Wednesday, April 9. "I have seen your beautiful face, heard your heartfelt words, and tasted my own tears crying for you and your family," Anne MacDowall of Burns Lake, British Columbia, e-mailed Barb. "It didn't take long for you to get inside me. It was time to quit. Smoking for 25 years, age 51. Thank you so much."

The flow of letters and e-mails had slowed. It had been six weeks since Barb's last school presentation. She worried that her message was fading away, but she believed she knew who to blame for that. "I'm pissed off at myself," she said. "There's no excuse."

The intravenous fluids continued to be more of a hassle than a help. Instead of hydrating her entire body, the fluids continued to gather at the injection site. If the site was in her arm, the arm would become bloated. The same happened with her back, chest, and, finally, her stomach.

"It just goes all over the place!" she told Tracy over the phone. "I'm so mad I could fucking scream. I just don't need this right now. This freakin' needle. I swear that nurse doesn't know how to put it in. They tried five times in five different sites!"

"Barb, I think it's your body," Tracy said. "I don't think it's the nurse."

"Well, there's got to be somebody who can put this in right."

"Why don't I take you to the Grey Nuns?"

"Are you kidding? If I go in there, they'll never let me out. I'm a palliative!"

A few hours later, though, Barb had calmed down. She joked with me over the phone that with the water build-up in her belly, she looked four months pregnant. "Actually, it was kind of cute. And I got to wear bigger jeans. I was excited."

She was no longer blaming the nurse. "It's just my body," she said. "It's my tissues."

Tracy also e-mailed me later in the day. Grub Med had been cancelled because of Pat's injury, but we all planned to meet the next day at the Delta Inn for a small birthday party.

"Barb said she is not cancelling tomorrow for nothing. Her nurses came in and now moved the I.V. needle from her stomach back to her arm vein. They needed it to go directly into the bloodstream because they have added three new drugs in her bags. I guess Barb went to hush up Halo, her psycho dog, when the nurse came in, and when she bent down to swat his nose, she fell over and the baby gate came off and she hit the floor and the nurse had to get her back up. She said she was so weak, she couldn't even help the nurse at all. Werner tells me Mackenzie is at our house for play and supper, which really, really surprises me as Barb doesn't let her out very often. Barb must really be feeling like crap and just wants to sleep."

Thursday, April 10. On Barb's 42nd birthday, Tracy, Craig Marler, Greg and I met her for lunch.

At long last, Barb was happy to report, her I.V. was paying off. "It's working. I've already gone through a full bag."

Barb also said she'd been drinking a lot of water, and had downed 60 ounces the previous day.

Just then, the waitress at the Delta recognized her. "The cameras don't do you justice at all."

"Thank you," Barb said, "even though I have three layers of make-up on my face, I appreciate that."

Greg brought Barb a rich chocolate cake from La Favorite, the city's top bakery. Barb gleefully blew out the candles.

Friday, April 11. Pat checked out of the hospital, and went straight to work. Later, he picked up a wheelchair for Barb. She again talked about speaking, bringing her chair and I.V. bags with her to be used as props. But Tracy wasn't so sure. She told me she doubted more than ever that another engagement would ever come off. "She still looks good to me, but I feel her more heavily leaning against me. When we get into the vehicle, she just slumps down low, and she just looks all shrunken."

Monday, April 14. "Everyone has a reason for being here," Geraldine Irlbacher Girtel of Edmonton e-mailed Barb. "Your purpose in this life goes beyond being a wife, mother, daughter, friend. You changed lives."

Barb had to cancel out on a school that morning. She'd been throwing up all night.

"She's been telling me for months the end is going to be awful, it's going to be awful," Tracy told me later that day. "It is awful now. As much as I'd like to think she's going to bounce back, I don't think she's going to do it."

But Barb wanted to keep booking schools. Donna Gingera lined up Louis St. Laurent, a large Edmonton junior high school, for later in the week.

Tracy had been given a copy of a CFRN documentary on Barb to pre-screen. In the video, Dr. Halperin said it was possible that Barb's crusade would save

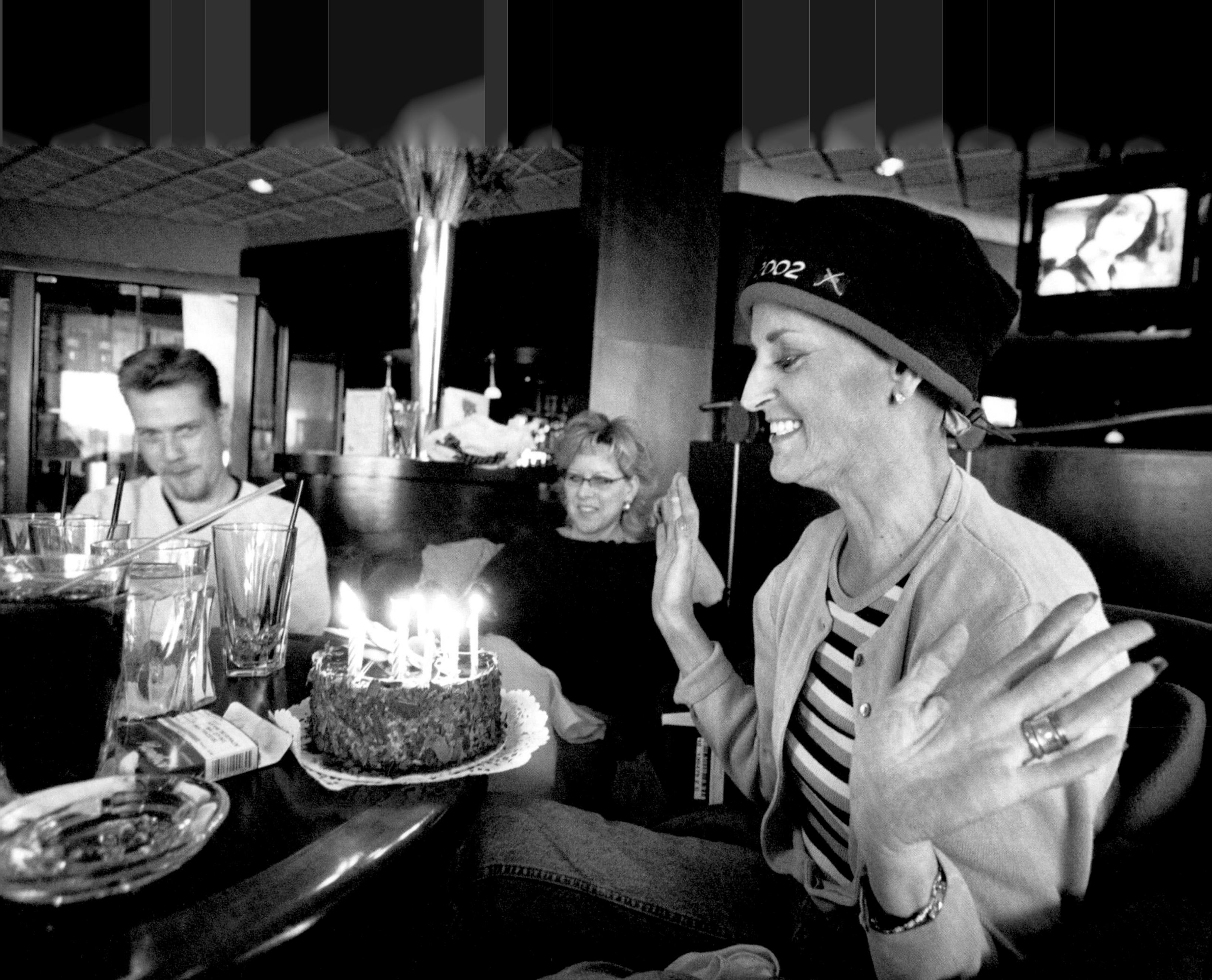

Barb celebrates her 42nd birthday on April 10 with Tracy and Craig Marler at the Delta Inn in south Edmonton

more people from lung cancer than he would in his career. As for her smoking, he said, "What I take away from that is, look at how difficult it is to quit smoking. Once you start, it's too late."

There was plenty of footage from earlier talks, including the massive shows in Red Deer, at the Jubilee and in Grande Prairie, where Barb had received standing ovations.

"It makes me realize, 'Holy shit, I was a part of all that,'" Tracy e-mailed me. "It makes me so proud to know her, so honoured to be a part of this with her."

In the evening, Barb was to appear on Al Stafford's CHED radio show. His studio was located on the station's second floor. There was no elevator. Stafford promised Tracy that, if needed, he'd carry Barb up the stairs.

"Bullshit!" Barb said when she heard of the offer. "I will walk up."

Rain poured down that evening. Barb wore a cream hat, cream sweater, white canvas pants, looking very sharp. She walked in on her cane. "You should see me in the wheelchair," she said. "I cruise! You know, in my first presentation, I said it doesn't matter if I'm blind, or in a wheelchair, nothing is going to stop me, the kids are going to see me. Well, that day is here. I'm going to come in on a wheelchair."

Stafford came down to the front door to meet Barb. He asked how Pat was doing. Barb said he was back in the hospital briefly, that after getting out, he'd gone right back to work, but was in a lot of pain. "My husband is a workaholic and he'll never change. It's Pat."

Barb then pulled herself up the stairs to the studio, Tracy supporting her by holding her arm.

On the air, Stafford teased her, "You stubborn Irish person, you had to walk up the stairs, didn't you?"

"Yeah, it took quite a while. I figure on the way down, I'll just sit down on the banister like I did when I was six or seven years old."

Barb then listed her severe symptoms. "The bottom line is, I'm at the end. I know it."

Her memory was gone, she said. People would say what day or what month it was, and she would be astonished to hear it was April. She wouldn't say anything, but would go and check the calendar and sure enough, it was April.

Her breath was now rattling in her chest. "That's a very common sound at the end of your life. But I'm not going to let it touch my spirit."

She told Stafford she planned to speak at Louis St. Laurent school later in the week.

"With all the work you've done, all the people you've met, haven't you done enough?"

"No, not at all. 'Cause this is what it does. Look at me."

"Are you ready to go?"

"I'm not afraid to go. I have no fear, not with my faith. . . I have strength I can't even explain."

Numerous callers phoned in to thank Barb. No more did anyone challenge her about her own smoking. After the show, Stafford helped Barb down the stairs. She leaned into him and smiled. "I use Tracy's body during the week," she said.

Barb came home to find an e-mail from Lynn DeCoste of Edmonton: "I can sit here and honestly say that there is no way that I could have had the fortitude to get out and speak to kids like you have. . . My mom always taught me growing up that the Lord never gives you more than He thinks you can handle, no matter how horrible it may be . . .You were selected for a reason, God's messenger if you will."

Tuesday, April 15. Barb had her belated birthday party at Grub Med. Two dozen friends and family showed up. She was in a festive mood. "I'm going to drink you under the table," she said to Werner, Tracy's husband.

I showed up with my three boys, Jack, Ned and Joe. Barb revelled in their presence, the sparkle she saw in them. I was thrilled they could meet her.

She stayed at the party for a few hours. She could manage just one bite of her lamb, a bit of potato and a few sips from her drink. In her usual fashion, she put a positive spin on it. "I had ice water," she later told me, "and that tasted the best of anything."

Wednesday, April 16. "When you first started to appear in the public eye, I was a little resentful and wondered why you chose to bring everyone down," Anny Krowko, a 22-year-old Edmonton woman, wrote to Barb. "Hey, if I am going to smoke, that's my decision, right? Well, no. I was wrong. Little did I know, I was affecting everyone I associated with. I made the decision to smoke, but my family, my pets, my friends, even strangers, were not given a choice. I made them smoke. I hate myself for that. I have been a non-smoker for 17 days now."

"You look great," Barb told Dr. Fonteyne at her check-up that day.

"So do you."

"Oh, liar, liar, pants on fire."

"How you feeling?"

"I feel lousy."

"Sleeping?"

"Seventeen hours a day, that's what I want to do. What do I do to stop sleeping so much?"

"You don't do anything. This is normal. You're going to be more tired as you get weaker. So just go with it. And if you get a lot of sleep, you'll be more alert in your waking hours."

"At least there's no diarrhea," Barb reported. "Very little. That's a reason to celebrate."

They both laughed.

She told Fonteyne about her I.V. problems and how her chest had inflated when the water pooled there.

"I became Dolly Parton, left side only."

"You're not walking that much?" Fonteyne asked.

"Yeah, I got my wheelchair."

"Where is it?"

"It's at home."

"That's a good place for it!" he scolded. "Use your wheelchair. Canes are bad. They're OK when you're feeling stronger, but when you're not strong, you can really take a fall. So use the wheelchair."

Barb wheezed when she tried to breathe in deeply.

"What do I do if my pulse drops?" she asked.

"Well, you don't have to do anything if it stops."

Again, they laughed. We all did, just like we did all the time now. Barb had always said she wanted life and laughter, and now she was getting a final heaping scoopful. It was so dark, what was happening to her, but she somehow made it light. Her spirit humbled me.

Thursday, April 17. Neither Barb nor Tracy had slept much through the night, anticipating the big event, Barb's talk at Louis St. Laurent. The bright, cold morning was like a gift. Barb felt fit to go, to do her first presentation in almost two months, her 46th public talk in all.

In the vehicle, Tracy glanced over at Barb. "Are you pumped?"

"Oh, am I!" she said, then was silent. When she spoke again, she was quiet. "You know what, though. I think this will be my last one."

"Oh, I don't know about that, Barb," Tracy said, still pumped up.

More than 1,200 teens packed into the gym. "Welcome Barb, we love you!" read a large poster on the wall.

The lights dimmed. Barb walked out, cane in hand. Images of her life projected onto the gym wall. Four TV cameramen followed her, illuminating her with their bright lights. In her red sweater and red hat, she looked like a lick of human fire.

Her performance was rambling, but coherent enough, as she updated the teens on her condition.

"The cancer has spread into the bones of my head!" she said in a loud, clear voice. "My head is going to get real bumpy and lumpy."

She'd lost 50 pounds now, she said, and collapsed all the time. She pointed to her wheelchair, which sat at the front of the gym. "The wheelchair is mine. I'm losing all my strength. Tell me, how cool is this? I walk down the street and I drop."

A few minutes in, Barb started to feel as if her legs would give out. She stopped walking around, leaned on her cane, and kept talking. "I have nausea and vomiting every day. Oh joy! I haven't thrown up in years. Now it's all I do."

Her hands shook as she spoke. "When you're having a hamburger or a hot dog or your favourite chocolate, think about this." She held up two empty intravenous bags. "This is what I have for breakfast, lunch and supper. My throat won't even let me swallow. This is what I eat. Is this a result, 100 per cent, of the smoking? You better believe it!"

Mackenzie's sweet face was projected on the wall. "My daughter Mackenzie is only 10. I'll never see her in junior high. I'll never see when she has a crush on a boy. I'll never see her when she wants to date, or wants to get married, or she has grandchildren. If you walk this path, it is full of pain. You have to say good-bye to the people you love."

She urged the students to help persuade their parents, friends and anyone else who smoked to quit.

"You could save their life," Barb said. "That's not exaggerating. *You could save their life!*"

The phrase stuck in my head. I had been hearing Barb say something similar since the start of her crusade. Now, however, there was no "if," attached to it, certainly not in her intonation. Barb knew she had done it, that she'd saved lives. All the children who had mobbed her, surrounded her and wept, all the broken cigarettes, all the letters, the promises from mothers, there could be no doubt. She didn't openly boast of her accomplishment, but I could hear the relief, satisfaction and excitement in her voice: "*You could save their life!*"

Just then, clarity came to me about the reason for all of this. It wasn't the obvious thing, it seemed to me, that Barb was a do-gooder, a hero, a saint. It wasn't

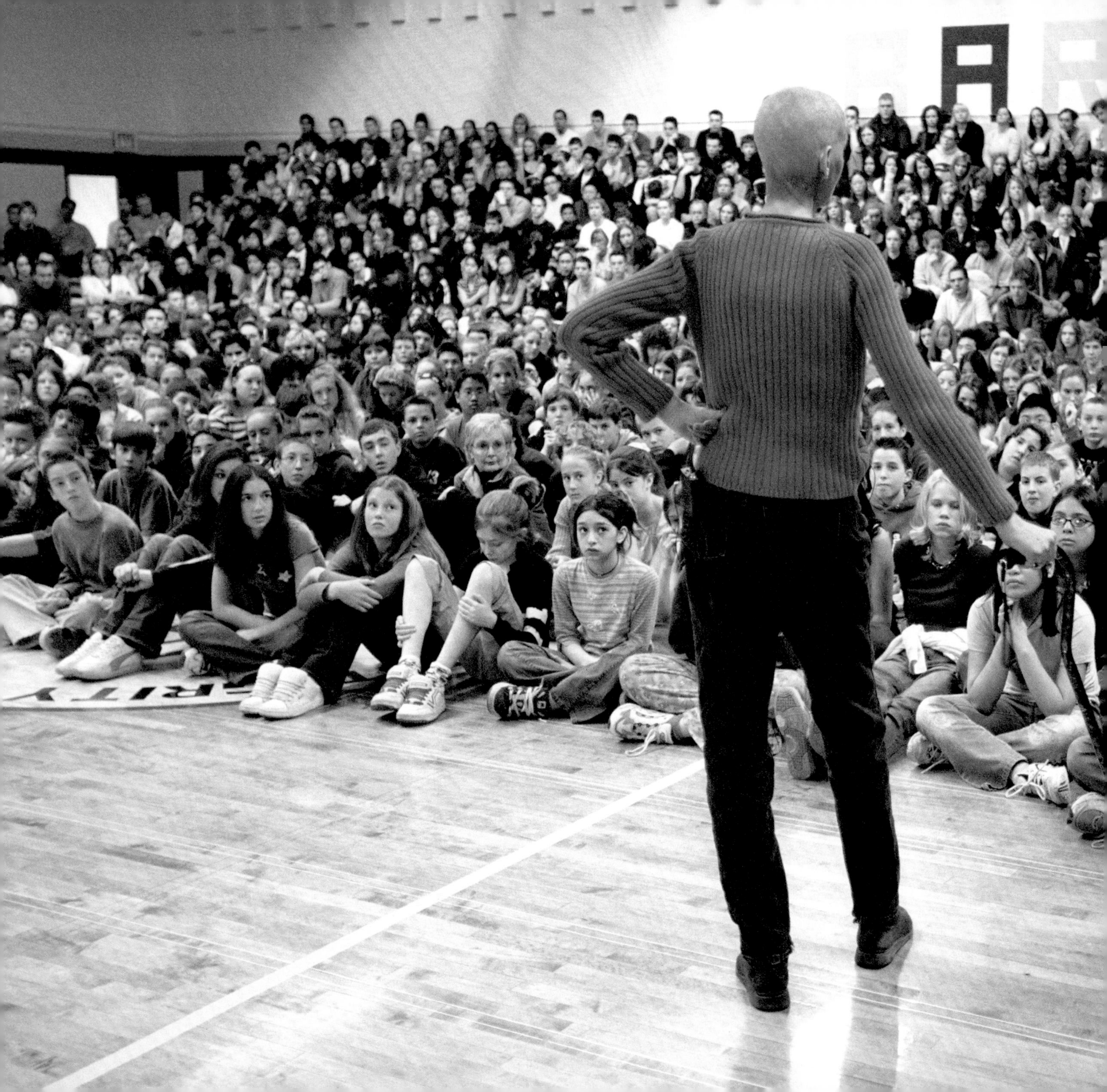

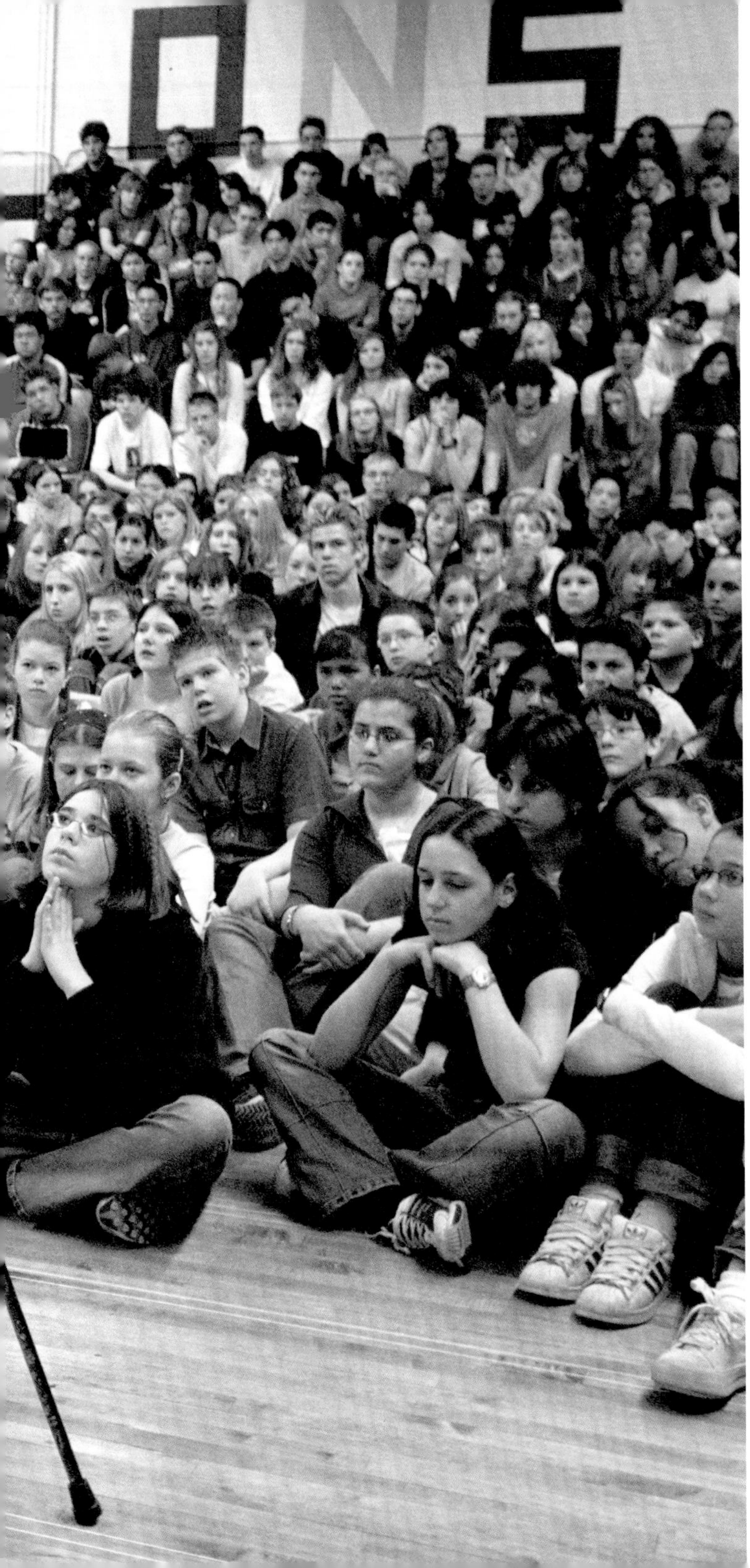

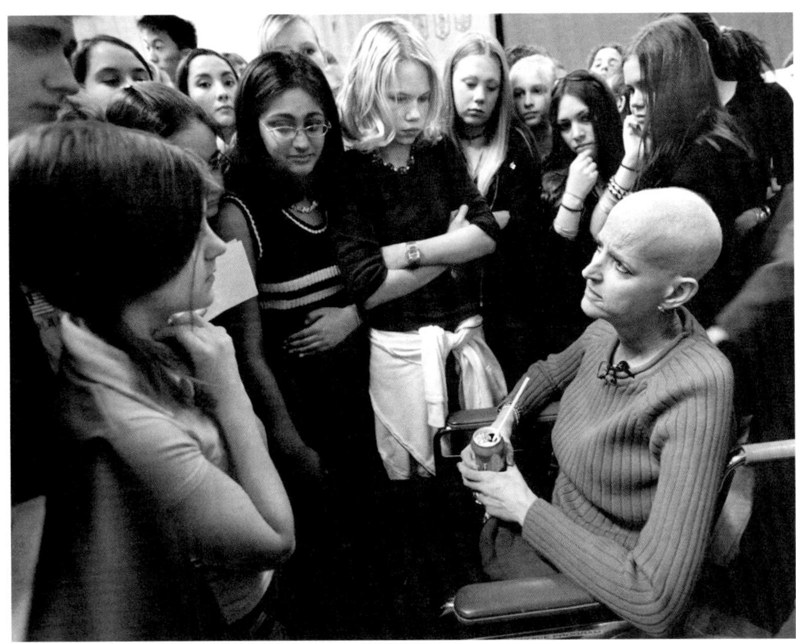

Barb listens to a group of students who surround her following her final talk, which was at Louis St. Laurent school on April 17. She was so tired after her presentation, she had to sit in her wheelchair. She used a cane during her presentation.

something that Barb ever talked openly about. It was about her loneliness.

I recalled the dozens of times I'd heard Barb talk about the pain of losing a loved one: her mom, her father, her twins. Not many, in safe and prosperous North America at least, know this kind of grief at such a young age as Barb did.

The destructive power of smoking had brought her unique anguish and isolation. It had created a void, a terrible loneliness, and loneliness was the great thirst for her, the hidden desert of her soul, parched and cracked, the hardest to quench.

Loneliness was especially hard to bear for a social butterfly like Barb. She craved companionship, friendship. Instead, she got the quiet of the house. Pat at work. Mackenzie at school. Herself. Her loneliness. Her cigarettes — oldest friends, oldest enemies.

She was a trouper, of course, with her spunk and blarney. She pushed down her loss and loneliness into a box and shut it tight. She never spoke of it. To some extent, I think, in her hard-headed way, she denied it. Still, it was there, hidden, explosive, ready for her to draw on in a moment when she needed to pull her tumour-ridden self up from the couch to speak at a school, or to rant at students, or to weep for the camera in an AADAC commercial. The pain was *right there.* And so was Barb's self-loathing.

She hadn't listened to Dr. Fields 20 years ago. She had smoked during her pregnancies. She had possibly smoked her twin boys to death. She had undoubtedly smoked herself to death.

As few others do, Barb understood death, and what her own passing would mean to Pat and Mackenzie. The loneliness that had pervaded her life was now going to be Mackenzie's fate. That longing for contact, for a talk, a laugh, a mother's hug, it was always going to be there.

Pat, he'd be OK. He was always OK. She wanted him to find a new love, a new life. But Mackenzie? Anxiety filled Barb, and that's why she was uncomfortable, always, with praise, with anyone calling her a hero, or a saint, or a crusader like Terry Fox. She knew the truth, I realized then.

She felt like a criminal.

Barb accepted that she had a great debt to pay, which is why she never got worked up about her own sickness and death. She knew she had those things coming. They were part of the payment.

And then, as if by chance, she found a way to make good. She could no longer embrace her mom, or little Patrick, or Michael, but she started to see them in everyone she met — and with every embrace, every interview, every talk, every standing ovation, every letter from a newly-minted non-smoker, a chunk of the debt was paid. That's why Barb was so crazy to get out there and speak, I realized. It was as if she was reaching into the future and changing things, giving years of precious life to men, women and children who otherwise would not have had them.

It was a tremendous gift to strangers, and, like so many good works, it rebounded back, in this case on Barb. She herself found a reward.

"*You could save their life!*"

Barb knew she had done it, she had saved lives, and it gave her an overwhelming sense that she'd paid her debt, that God had forgiven her. Her crusade filled the lonely places inside. It healed her. At the end of her life, ravaged by decay and pain, pumped full of morphine, anti-seizure drugs and steroids, she had reconciled herself to her past. She atoned for her life's great mistake. She was able to move on.

The huge crowd of students at Louis St. Laurent stood and cheered for Barb. Afterwards, well-wishers swamped her. In the crush, she found it hard to breathe. Tracy and Craig Marler rushed in with her wheelchair so she could sit, regain her balance. She was exhausted, but those around her were ecstatic.

"That was great!" said Tracy to me, glowing now. "She did really, really well. She missed this."

Barb's performance at the school had reminded all of us that we'd been given a rare opportunity to work closely with a person of extraordinary conviction. Even Little Barb, a heavy smoker herself who had small use for Barb's crusade, was impressed. "I have no idea how she did it," she told me afterwards. "When I saw her the week before, she literally couldn't talk. She wasn't walking at home, she was using her wheelchair. But she pulled it together."

Saturday, April 19. Montel Williams and his research team sent Barb a dozen white roses as a belated birthday gift. "It made Barb's day," Tracy told me. "They are absolutely gorgeous."

Easter Sunday, April 20. Pat offered to get Barb into her wheelchair to go for a walk with Mackenzie, but Barb had no inclination to get off the couch. She stayed under an electric blanket. Even there, she felt cold. Her feeling of exhaustion never left her now. She threw up relentlessly, wave after wave of dry heaves. For the first time, she didn't put on her makeup.

Pat looked downhearted when Tracy dropped by in the afternoon. Barb told Tracy she didn't think she would make it through the weekend.

"This sucks," she said. "I hate it."

Pat made a turkey for Easter dinner. Barb tried some Jell-O, but threw it all up. Even the smell of the turkey made her feel like vomiting, but she didn't complain. She told Tracy how grateful she was that Pat had put in the effort.

Just then, it flashed through Tracy's mind how kind and friendly Barb had been through most of her illness. Tracy felt humbled, the same as I had felt.

"I've learned a lot in the last six months about how to treat people and just give it your all, because everybody is so special," she e-mailed me.

In some ways, though, this made Tracy hurt all the more. "I'm getting really scared. I find myself thinking about getting a phone call and rushing out the door to see Barb. I can't believe this is really happening. Everybody thinks I'm so strong and coping well. I think on the inside I'm pretty much a basketcase. I don't want Barb to go. I will miss her so much. As I cry myself to sleep, I think about what she must be thinking. I can't imagine."

Monday, April 21. "You have gotten MANY of my friends to quit smoking," Kirsten McGinn, a student at Louis St. Laurent, e-mailed Barb. "I promise you, I will never smoke another day. I have tried and it is gross."

I had to travel to Brandon, Manitoba, to cover a murder trial, a case I'd been involved in for some time. I hated being away, but I had no choice.

Tuesday, April 22. Barb rarely answered her phone, but Tracy got through at lunch time. They talked briefly, then Barb said, "Well, I'm just going for a nap, 'cause I haven't had one."

"Oh yeah. What did you do all morning?"

"Well," Barb said, "I slept."

They both laughed.

In the moments when Barb was awake and alert, she didn't want to miss a thing that was going on, so she sacked out on the couch in the living room, not the bedroom.

"Her voice is still up," Tracy e-mailed. "It's not a depressed, down, awful voice."

Wednesday, April 23. Tracy talked to Pat, who said Barb was barely eating, just some pudding a few days back and a few bites of Kentucky Fried Chicken. She was on her daily maximum of morphine, which made her very sleepy, though she constantly had to get up to go to the toilet. Each time, Pat had to haul her up into her wheelchair. He was becoming exhausted.

Thursday, April 24. Tracy again found Barb to be confused when she got her on the phone.

"I'm waiting for the guys," Barb said.

"What guys? You have guys coming over?"

"Well, it's the end of the month. You know the school kids. The lights are on and everything is unglued."

"What are you saying?"

"What?"

"You want me to come over? I think you're talking funny like you did before."

"They'll be here right away."

Barb then became more coherent. She said she just needed a nap. Her big hope, she told Tracy, was to have Dr. Fonteyne take her off her anti-seizure medications, which she was certain were responsible for her grogginess.

Friday, April 25. Barb was too tired to go to Dr. Fonteyne's office. Pat and Tracy went instead. They told Fonteyne about Barb's desire to go off her medications.

"She thinks they're making her feel like crap," Tracy said.

"Certainly she can go off the medications," Fonteyne said. "I can't tell her what to do. She's always got that option. The problem is if she goes off the Decadron, for example, the brain is going to swell more, she's going to have more pain, more neurological signs, probably her rate of seizures will go way up."

"And she really hasn't had any for two months," Pat said.

"She could go off those things and conceivably nothing would happen," Fonteyne said.

"But doubtful," Pat said.

"Yeah, and the other medications she's taking are not giving her any problems."

"For some reason she believes the medication is what makes her tired," Pat said.

"It's the progression of the cancer. Cancer takes a lot out of you. It steals your energy. It takes your nutrition away. This is what happens."

"Should she be in palliative care?" Tracy asked.

"That's my question for you guys," Fonteyne said. "What have you talked about so far? Would you like her in palliative care?"

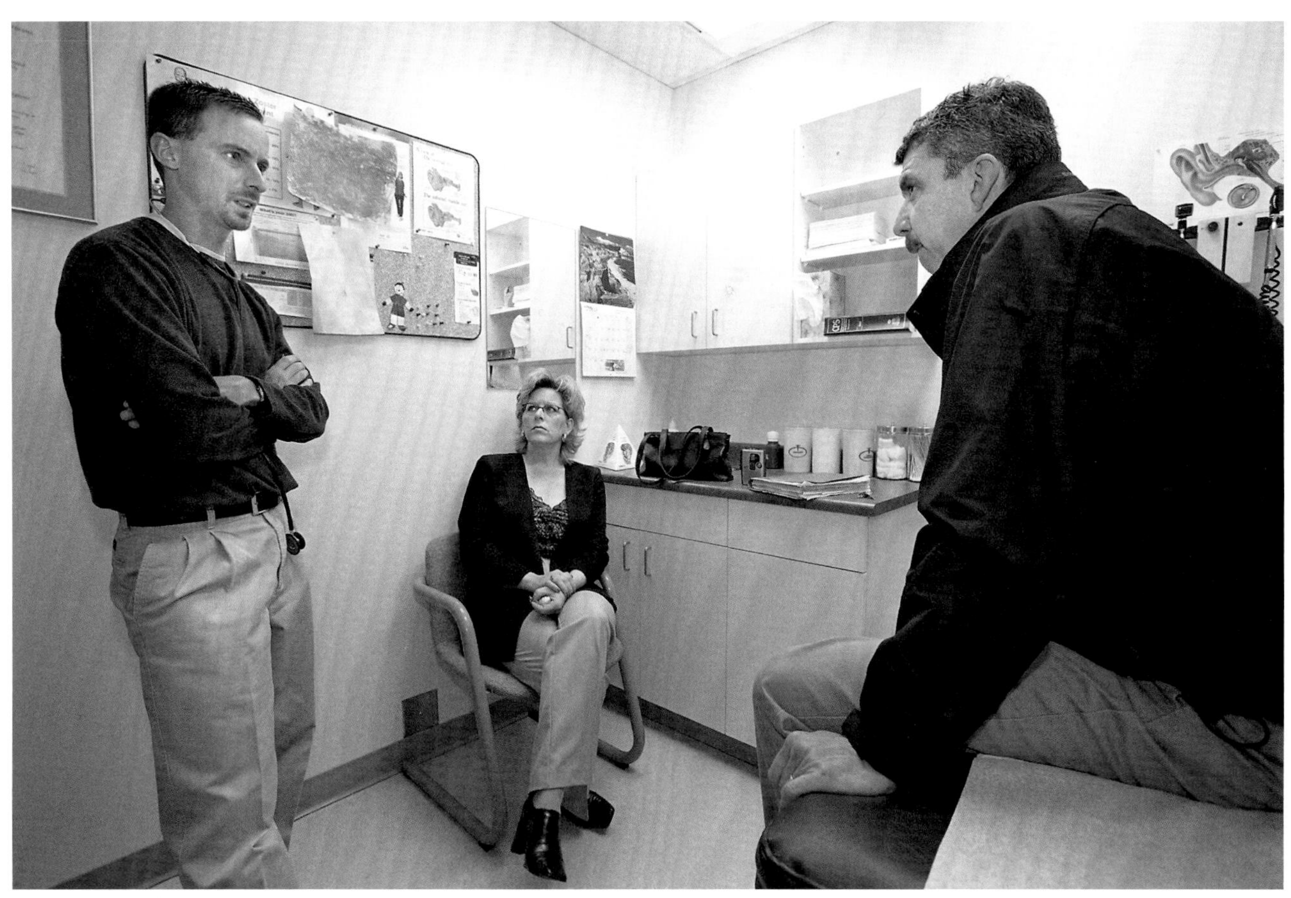

The debate over Barb's future: Dr. Fonteyne, Tracy, and Pat.

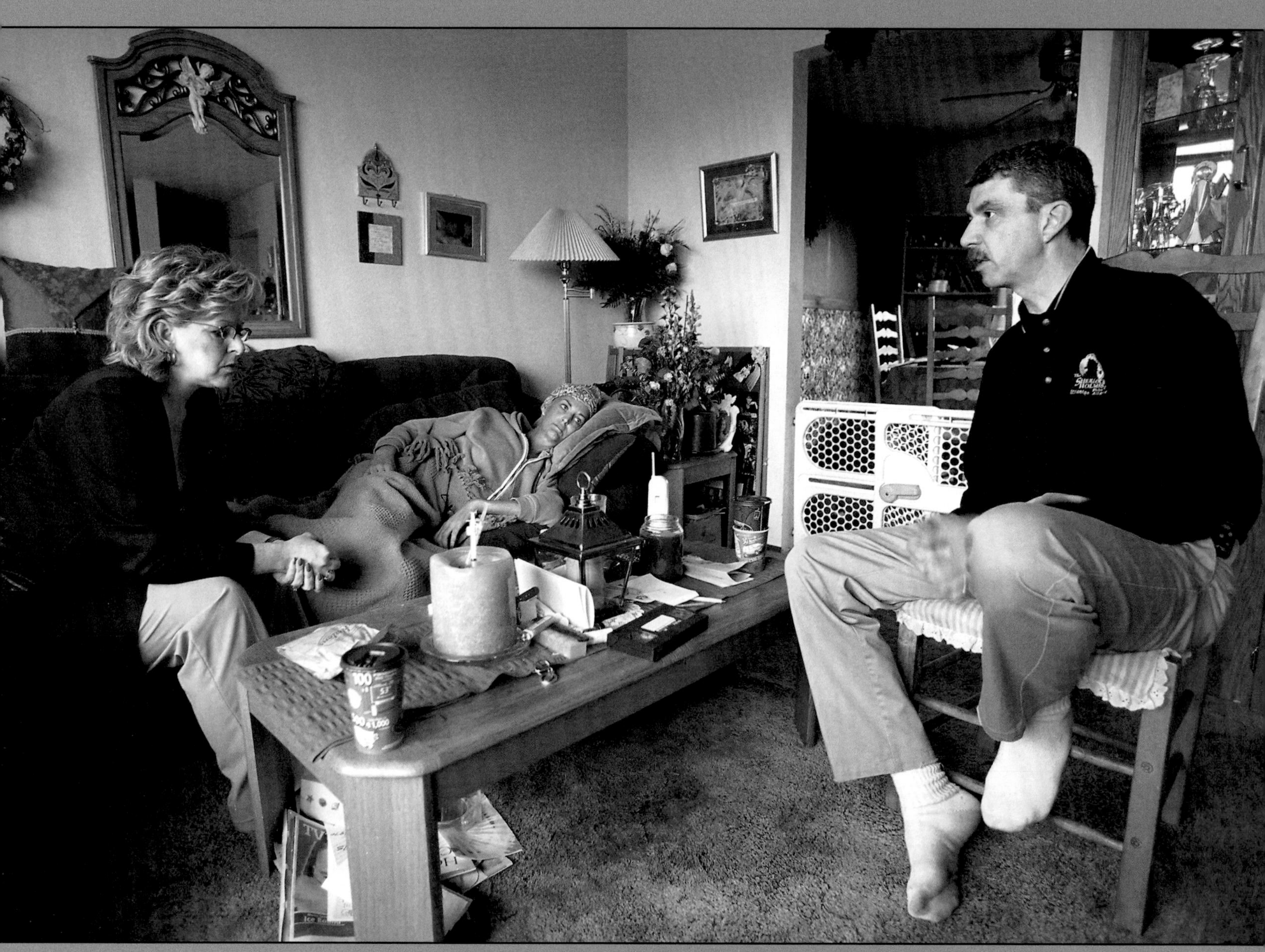

Pat and Tracy talk to Barb after meeting with Dr. Fonteyne.

"I think she's leaning that way," Pat said.

Fonteyne said he would arrange for a home-care doctor to visit Barb and Pat later that day to help them make a decision.

"So she shouldn't go off the medication?" Tracy asked to conclude.

"I don't want her off anything," Fonteyne said.

Pat and Tracy returned to the Tarbox home to pass the news on to Barb. She lay on the couch, looking like an old crone, sunken cheeks, shrivelled lips sucked in around her teeth, a vacant hole for a mouth. Pat and Tracy told her what Fonteyne had said.

"He's just worried that going off the meds will make it worse," Tracy said.

"OK?" Pat said.

Barb scowled. "So all I can do, I can't walk. I just lie here?"

"Going off medicine, Barb, is not going to make you well," Pat said.

"So I don't walk?"

"It's just at that stage, Barb. He said it's best for the progression of the cancer."

Barb continued to scowl.

"It's not what you wanted to hear, is it?" Tracy said.

"I don't know what you thought going off the drugs was going to do," Pat said. "Fonteyne doesn't prescribe something because he wants to. He does it because it's good for you, sweetie. You know that."

"I don't want to be so sleepy," Barb said at last.

"The meds aren't making you sleep, Barb," Pat said. "You've eaten a tub of Jell-O in four days. It's that cancer that gives you no appetite."

In the evening, a home-care doctor told Barb that in palliative care they would take her off all her medications, clean out her system, then start her up again with new medications. It was possible she would rebound and be out of the hospital in a week to 10 days.

Maybe there was something they could do after all, Barb and Pat both thought.

Saturday, April 26. Barb continued to be cranky, Tracy e-mailed me in Brandon. "Everything Pat says or does, she gets pissed off. He can't do anything right at this point . . . A person usually lashes out at the ones closest to them."

Monday, April 28. Barb got up at 5 a.m. to put on her makeup in preparation for checking in to Unit 43, the 14-bed palliative care ward at the nearby Grey Nuns hospital. Donna Gingera had issued a press release about the move, and Barb knew there would be reporters and cameramen at the hospital.

Tracy picked up Barb at 8:20 a.m. She still looked great, Tracy thought.

"Let's do our thing," Barb said.

They headed off, just like old times, stopping in at a coffee shop to pick up a coffee, a Coke and a newspaper.

At the hospital, Barb answered a few questions from the throng of reporters. She told everyone she would be in for a few days, a week at most. As soon as she was alone with Tracy and Pat, Barb turned to Tracy and said, "Your mission is to find a smoking room."

"Well, we might have to go downstairs."

"No," interjected Pat, who had already spied Unit 43's smoking lounge. "How about just ten feet away?"

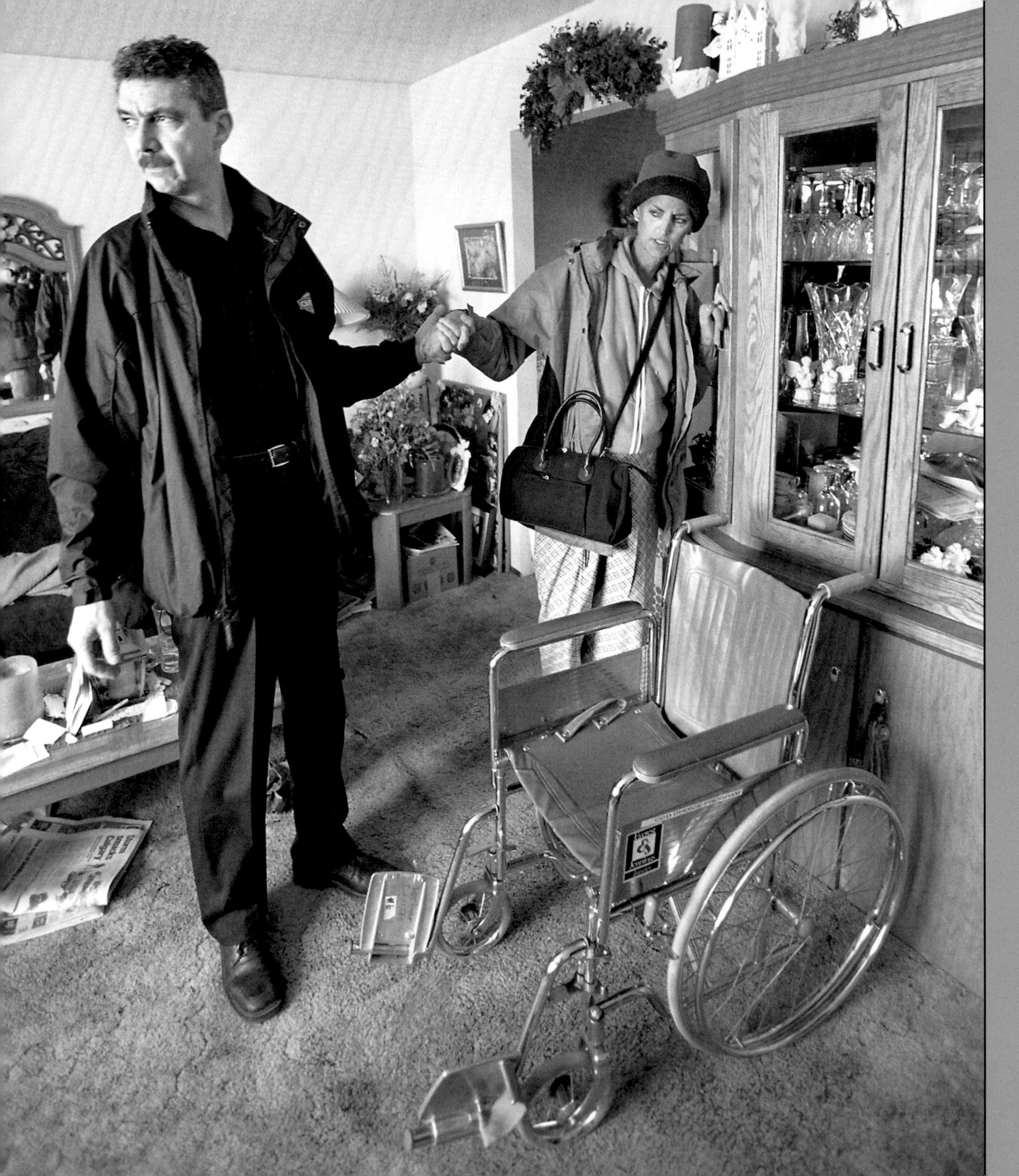
Storm
smacks
Calgary

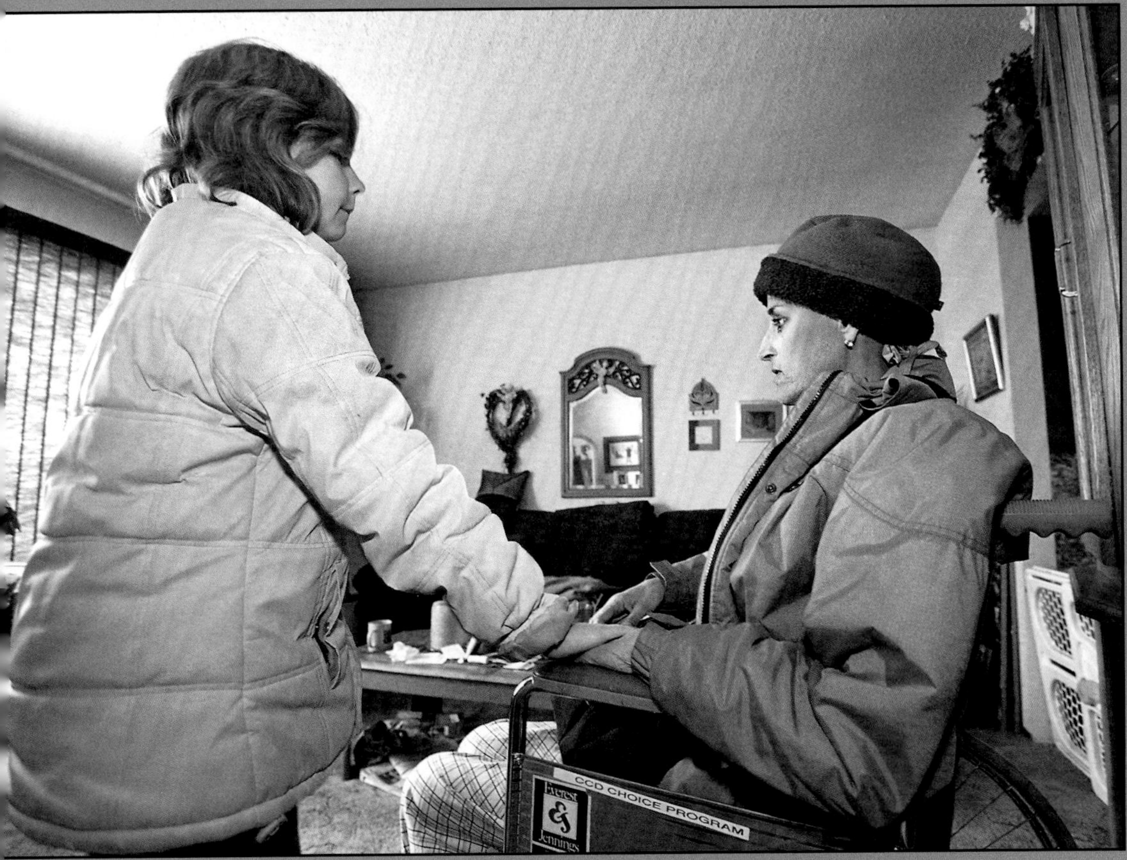

Mackenzie says goodbye to Barb and leaves for school. This is the last time she will see her mother at home.

Opposite page: Pat helps Barb into her wheelchair as they leave their home to admit Barb into the palliative care ward.

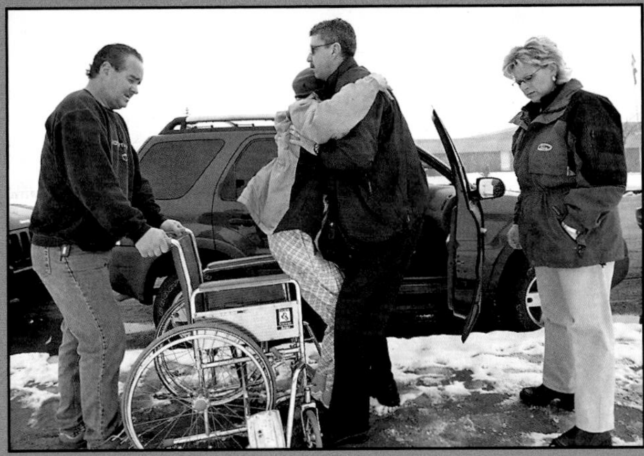

Werner Mueller holds onto Barb's wheelchair as Pat helps Barb.

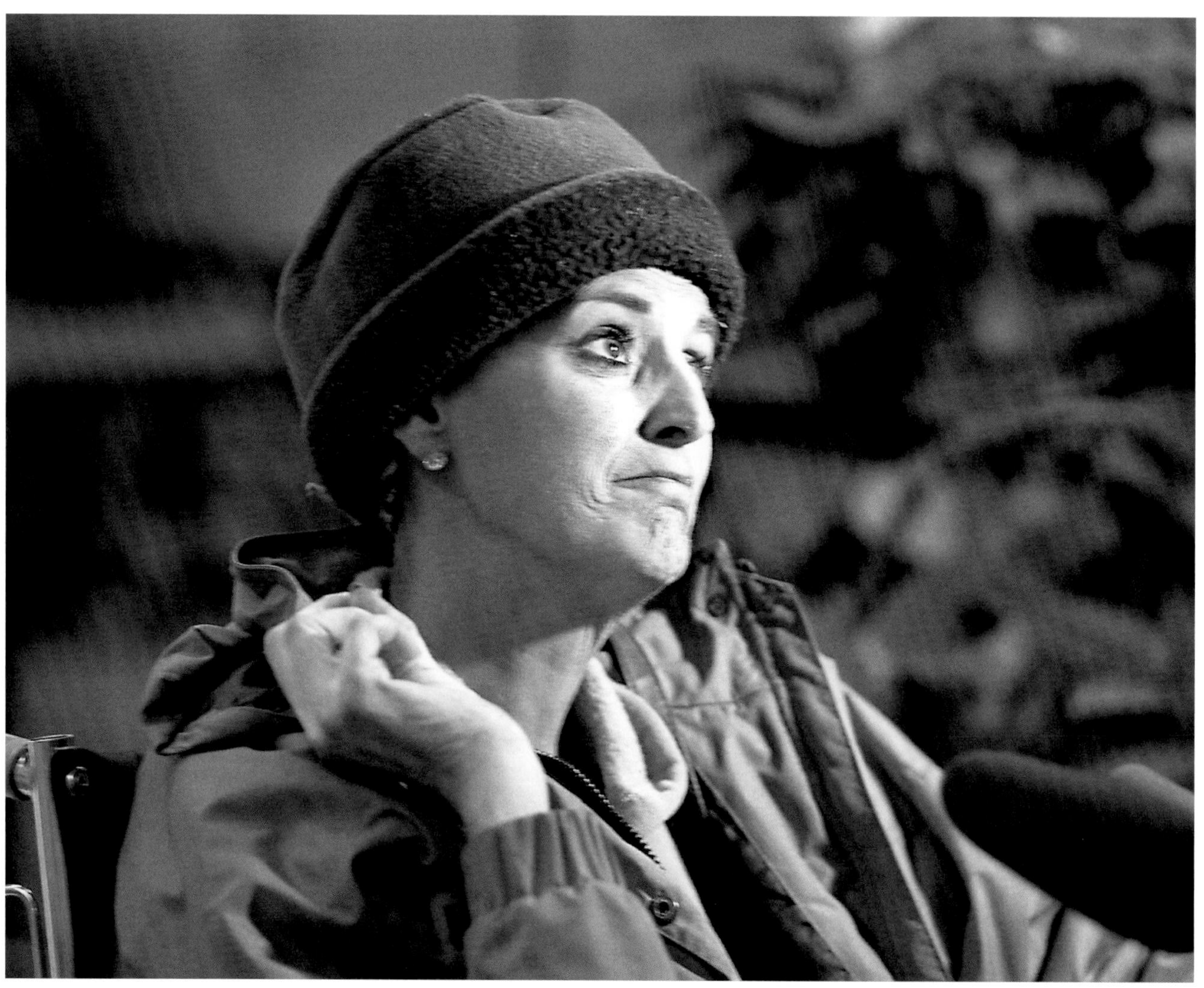

Barb gives her final press conference just outside the palliative care ward before being admitted into the hospital.

Right away, Barb went in for a smoke. "This is the greatest place in the world," she said.

Her first impression wasn't lasting, however. The lounge was a sad place.

The door to the room was always closed. A sign on it read: "Only Patients From Unit 43 Allowed To Smoke In This Room." In the early 1990s, administrators had decided the hospital must be smoke-free, that staff and patients alike had to smoke outdoors. An exception was made for Unit 43. The dying were deemed too feeble to make the lengthy journey along two hallways, down an elevator and through the main lobby to smoke outside.

Chilly air flowed through the lounge to vent the fumes, but a stale cigarette odour remained. There was no TV, no radio, no board games, no comfortable furniture. It was all business, all addiction maintenance: go in, light up, smoke, back to bed.

Patients shuffled in or got pushed in on wheelchairs. Some of them were so weak and drugged up, they nodded off and dropped their lit cigarettes. Dozens of burn marks, the colour of yellowy-brown nicotine-stained fingers, scarred the linoleum floor and cheap furniture. Barb grew agitated when she saw the marks, not knowing quite what they were. "We've got to do something about this."

"It's burn marks," Tracy said.

Barb looked disgusted. "What's wrong with people?"

"They fall asleep, Barb. If there's nobody in here, the cigarette drops."

"It's driving me crazy. Clean that up."

Tracy covered over the marks around Barb by placing a blanket under her wheelchair. Tracy also decorated Barb's room, putting up photographs of Barb's friends on a bulletin board, arranging cards and flowers.

The room had a window, a bed, a TV, a VCR and a stereo, the electronics all donated by the families of previous patients.

In her initial check-up, Barb outlined her symptoms to Dr. Paul Mendosa, telling him how her vision had gone from 20/20 to 20/270, her appetite had disappeared, and she had lost 80 pounds. "My mother had lung cancer," she said. "I know what is coming. It's OK. It's OK. But there comes a point where I don't want to be at home. You hear my chest? I feel like a rattle. I don't want my ten-year-old to see me die at home."

"How do you describe your pain?" Mendosa asked.

"It is inhuman. I've never felt this kind of pain in my life. It's sharp and it stays there. It doesn't move off."

He asked if she was having any unusual or vivid dreams.

"Oh yeah. Hallucinations. That's me. I swear."

Barb was taken off oral morphine and started to get injections, quadrupling her intake of the drug.

Hospitals are known to be leery of newspaper photographers, especially in light of doctor-patient confidentiality rules. Barb had put Greg and me on a list of people who were to be allowed into her room, but Greg didn't know how the medical staff would accept him. As Barb settled in, he started to take photographs. A nurse gave him a look, which Barb noticed.

"Don't worry," she said. "That's just my wee brother."

"Oh, he's your brother."

"No, he's not my real brother. He's a photographer."

Greg jumped in, explaining to the nurse what he was doing, documenting Barb's entire story. For the time being, things seemed OK.

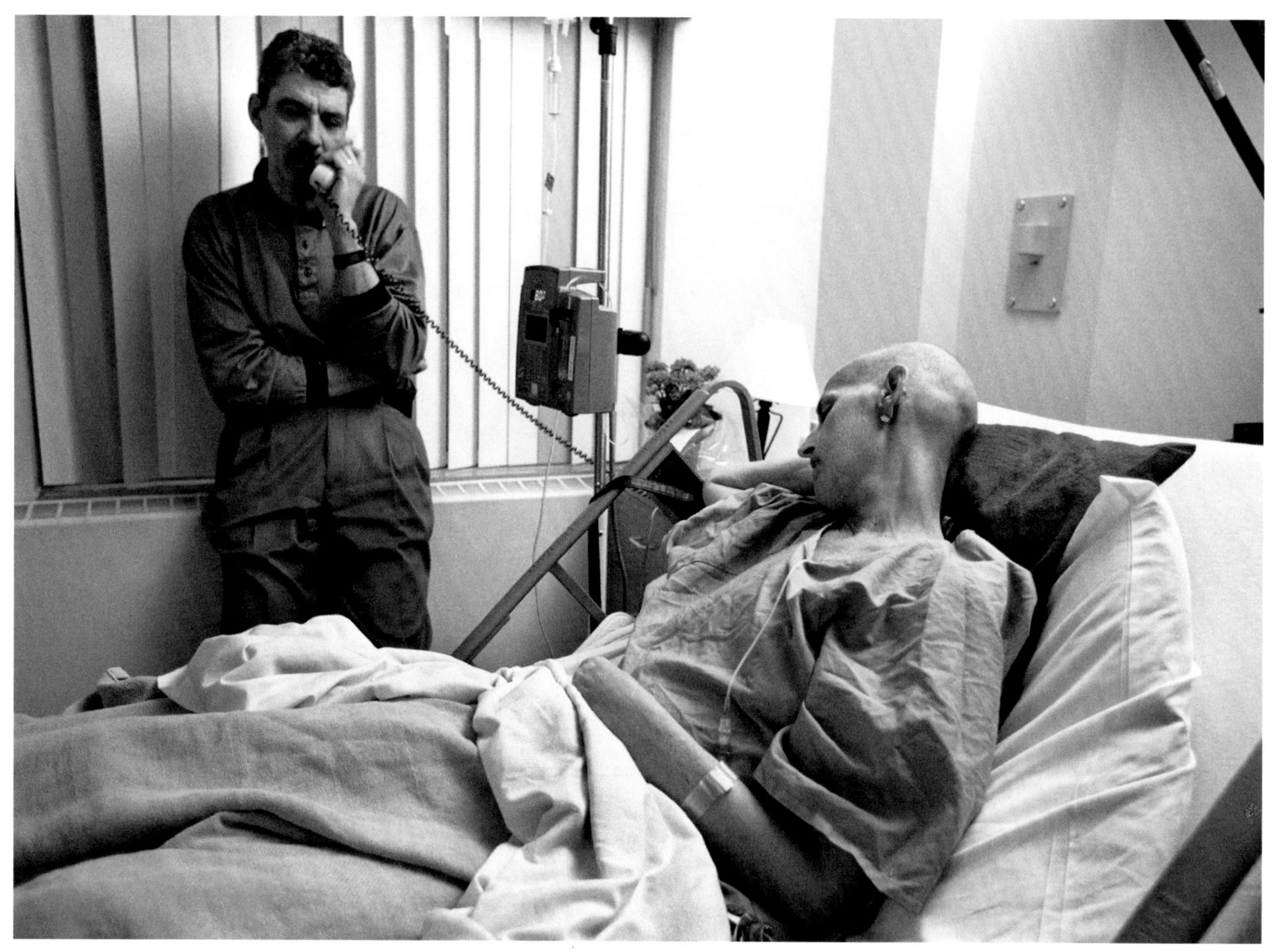

Barb's first day in palliative care. Pat says good night to Mackenzie, who is staying with Little Barb.

Tuesday, April 29. Tracy came in that morning and found that Barb already had on make-up, in anticipation of a short visit from Mayor Bill Smith.

"Somebody put on your make-up?" Tracy asked.

"No."

"You put it on?"

"No."

"Barb, somebody put make-up on you."

"Oh yeah," Barb said and laughed. "I remember. I did."

When Mayor Smith visited, she was her old, upbeat self, saying, "Well, you know, Mayor, I'm not done yet."

For the remainder of the day, she did little but sleep, fading in and out of consciousness. Her new regime of medications appeared to have knocked her out.

Now and then, she asked to go for smoke breaks, but barely inhaled.

"She doesn't even want it," Tracy e-mailed me. "Even when she's having one, it's more habit. She doesn't smoke it. She just holds it. She's too tired."

Barb's unending, delirious sleep so worried Tracy and Pat that at one point they considered asking her priest, Father Mike Mireau, to give her the last rites. Greg was anxious as well. The burden of his responsibility to photograph Barb on her deathbed kept him at the hospital for endless hours. Even when Pat, Tracy and Barb's other friends and family had left, he remained. But he took no more photographs. He found he could not lift up his lens.

Barb was so helpless, Greg thought. It was scary to watch her. She would wake up, look around in a fog, not know where she was, then conk out again.

At one point, Barb sat slumped over, a tube in her nose. Greg saw this was a strong image, the kind of shot that Barb had always talked about, an ugly, graphic picture of a smoker's death. Greg was all alone in the room, no one else around, no nurses to watch him. He could easily have taken the shot without anyone knowing it. But he did not.

He made sure to keep the door of Barb's room open. He didn't want any nurse coming in and accusing him of being a media vulture, of secretly snapping pictures of her.

Tracy printed out a bunch of e-mails from Barb's mailbox. When she showed up at the hospital in the evening, she read them to Barb. Barb may or may not have heard them, Tracy didn't know, but she read them just in case. One came from Jaime Hurl of Edmonton, who was 26 years old and had been smoking since she was 12. She'd often tried to quit smoking, but to no avail until she heard Barb. "I remember hearing you say that you would like to see your daughter grow up," Tracy read to Barb. "Well, I have decided I would like to live to eventually have mine."

Wednesday, April 30. Again, Greg camped out at Barb's bedside. Again, he had his camera, but was unable to lift it. Barb lay as lifeless as ever, but she no longer had the tube in her nose. This unmistakeable visual sign of illness and death was no longer available to be photographed. Greg berated himself for missing the shot. For all he knew, Barb would soon die, and he would have missed the single most compelling image of her last moments at the hospital.

Later that afternoon, however, the tube went back in.

This is where Barb is at, Greg told himself. *You've*

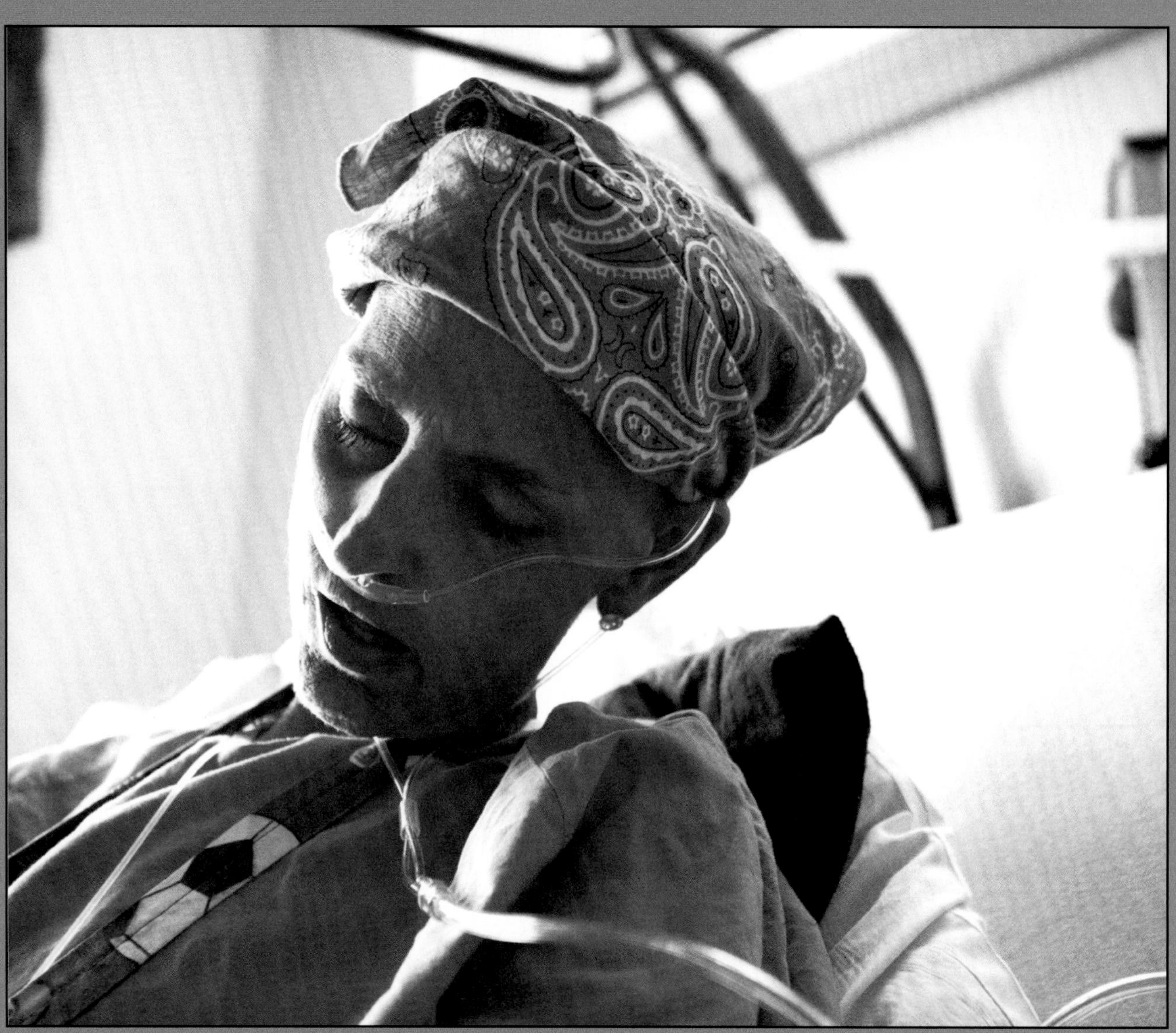

got to do it. You have to grab your camera and you have to start taking pictures.

Still he sat.

I can't. I cannot do it.

He realized then what was wrong, that he feared the judgment of others, that they might see him taking these pictures and they would think something was wrong with him, that he was an uncaring man. But this just wasn't true. He was Barb's friend.

Greg thought back to what Barb had always said. She wanted the ugliest pictures possible. He had promised to take them. He had spent the last six months doing the groundwork, making sure he was close enough to Barb that he would be in this position now.

You have got to come through.

He picked up his camera. He started shooting.

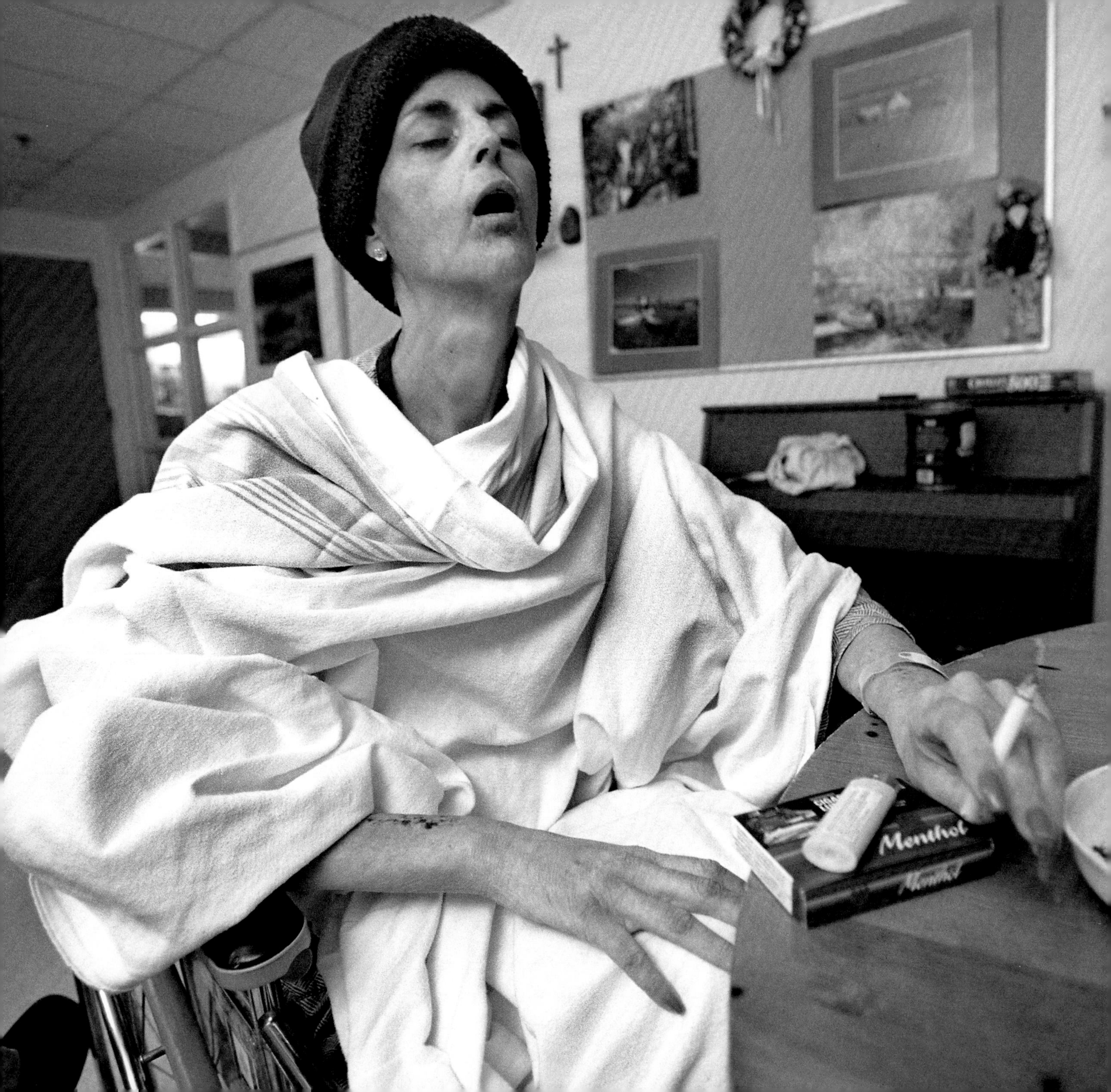
Menthol
Menthol

May

2 0 0 3

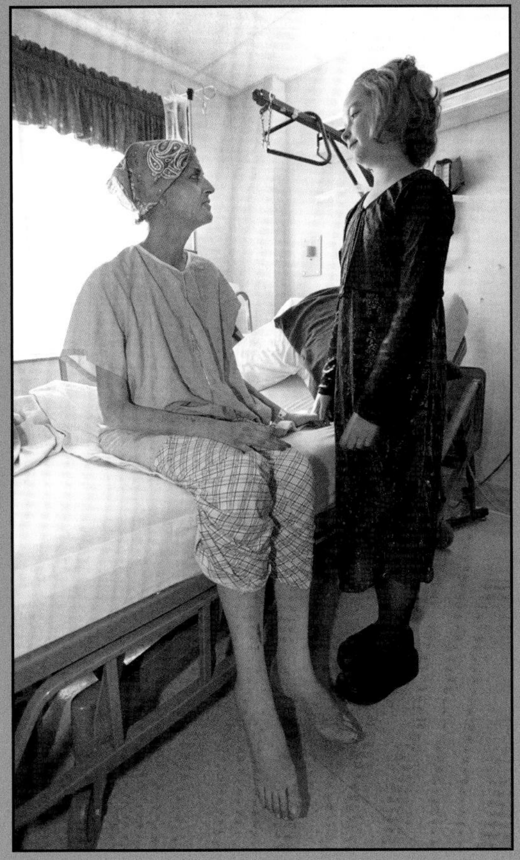

Time held me green and dying
Though I sang in my chains like the sea.

Dylan Thomas

Thursday, May 1. Tracy visited in the morning and was astonished to see Barb awake and alert, her make-up on. Barb seemed to be adjusting to her new medication regimen, which meant she was much more active, and wanting to get up to smoke.

She couldn't lift herself up from the bed, so each time she wanted to smoke, the person helping her would go through the same ritual: turn off and unhook her I.V. drip, move Barb's legs off the bed, pull Barb up to sitting position, count down with her, *three, two, one*, lift her off the mattress, direct her into the wheelchair. She often landed hard. Her urine bag was unhooked from the bed and hung on a hook on her wheelchair. She would get wheeled into the smoking lounge, light up, have a few puffs, then go back to bed. She would sleep 15 or 20 minutes, then the process would repeat itself.

In the lounge, she would often fumble with her lit cigarette, hitting her chin, her upper lip, before finally getting it into her mouth. Once, she dropped a burning smoke into her lap.

"Ah! Ah! Ah!" she yelped, before Tracy flipped her gown, shooting the cigarette into the air.

At one point, Tracy asked her, "Is it habit that you need to come in here or do you crave a smoke?"

"I don't know," Barb said wearily, shaking her head, fed up with the focus on her continued smoking, and beyond caring about giving a contrite, politically correct answer. At last, she told the truth, what she'd been thinking all along when people questioned her about her habit.

"Shut up," she told Tracy.

Tracy and Pat worried that Barb might be tiring herself out with her restless treks to the smoking lounge.

"Let's go to the smoke room," she pestered Pat at one point. "Let's go to the smoke room."

"Nah," Pat said. "Sweetie, you got to get some rest."

"Well, I got to go to the bathroom."

With that, Pat got her up. When she went towards the bathroom, however, she slammed shut the door without going in.

"OK," Barb said triumphantly. "*Now* let's go for a smoke."

Greg made sure to take numerous pictures of Barb smoking. At one point, she looked at him snapping away and made a wry smile, as if she knew what a ridiculous and pitiful image she presented, and that was just the way she wanted it.

Friday, May 2. A core group of friends and family — Pat, Tracy, Little Barb, Pat's mom Giselle Tarbox, and Barb's friend Susan Shaw, who used to teach Michael at school — started to take turns caring for her around the clock. Giselle, whom everyone called Mrs. T., took the morning shift. Little Barb was there in the afternoon, until Tracy or Susan Shaw would relieve her in the evening. Pat came and sat through the night with her. When Barb woke up, there was always someone there now.

That day, the court case in Brandon slowed down, and I was able to return to Edmonton. I was so thankful and relieved that Barb was still alive. On my way home from the airport, I dropped in to see her.

She looked alert, better than I had expected. Pat told me she'd eaten a few bites of scrambled egg and had some coffee, which gave him hope that she might

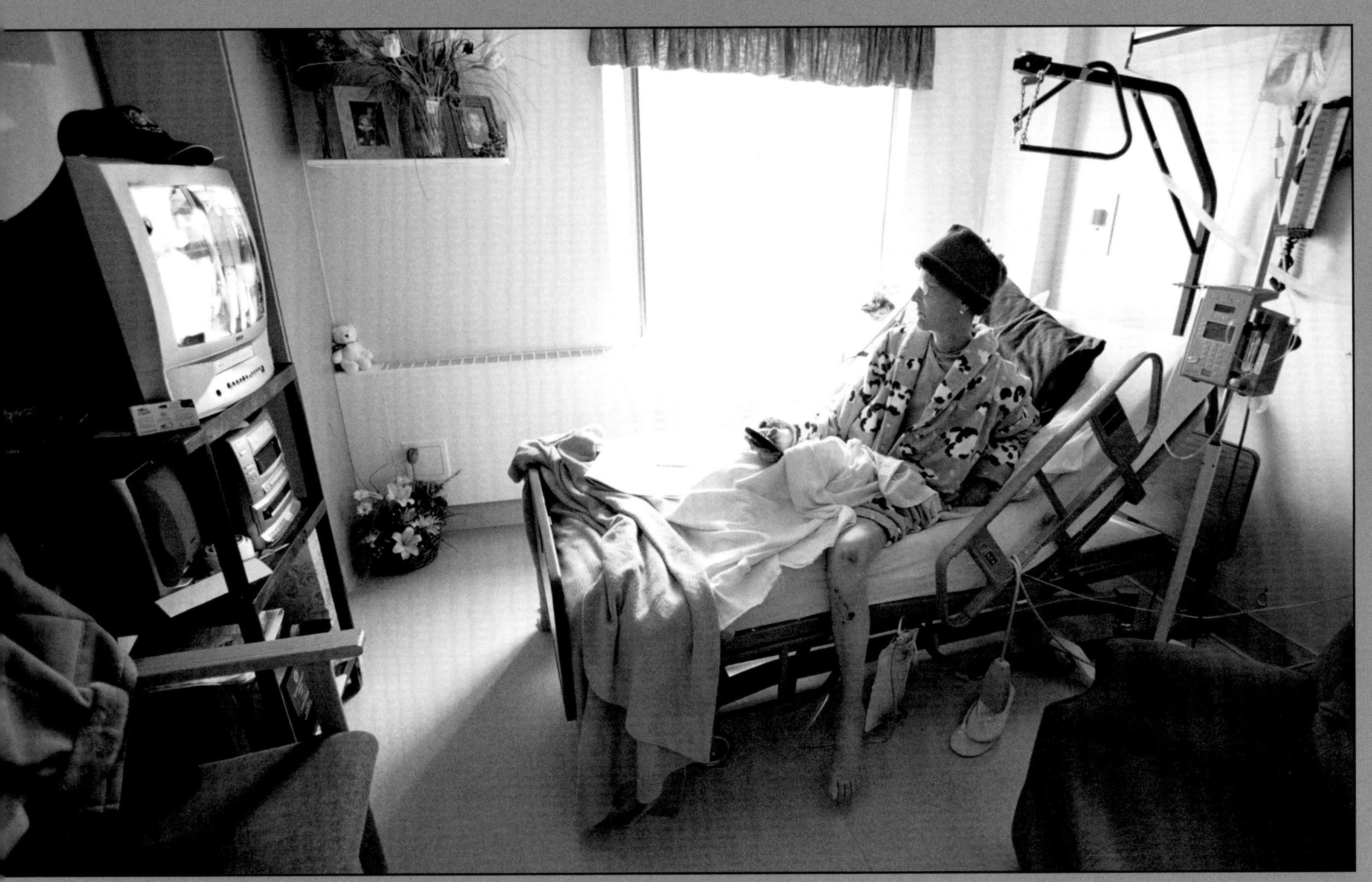

improve after all, and be well enough to go home. It was the first time she'd eaten in five days.

Tracy's boss from Team Ford, Neil Reid, dropped by. "You're looking a lot better," he told Barb.

"I feel really out of it," she said.

"That's because you finally are able to complain that you're out of it," Pat said. "On Tuesday and Wednesday you slept 23 out of 24 hours. So to say you're feeling that way is pretty amazing, and to eat something is phenomenal."

That afternoon in the smoking lounge, Little Barb noticed the ash was going to fall off Barb's cigarette and burn her housecoat. "You want me to flick your ash? I'll flick it before it falls on your housecoat."

"Move your fence," Barb said.

Little Barb turned to me and said, "When she's talking about, 'Move my fence,' she's talking about something else. But she wants you to move something."

Later, as she lay in bed, Barb said, "I need the dryer. Who's turning their car?"

Then: "OK, what did I do with that *eran*?"

"The *eran*?" Tracy asked her, holding up Barb's denture plate.

"No, not that," Barb said.

Tracy kept searching, determined to go through every item in the room if that's what it took to get Barb what she wanted. At last, Tracy handed over the TV remote.

"Yes," Barb said and smiled.

"*That's* the *eran*," Tracy said. "I'll remember that."

Saturday, May 3. The TV was almost always on in Barb's room. The sound comforted her. She would perk up whenever she heard one of her AADAC commercials come on.

Just before noon, Father Mike Mireau visited.

"So how are you doing today?"

"Not bad," she said sleepily, her speech slurred. "It's just because I did that."

"Are you peaceful?"

"Yeah." Barb's eyes were barely open.

"Very peaceful."

"They made you strong, didn't they?"

"Yeah."

"You've done good work."

"I take the wipetail out," Barb said, and mumbled a few more sentences, looking very grave.

"We all make mistakes," Father Mike said, guessing her meaning. "But God can forgive us of our mistakes and make good things out of them. And He did that with you."

Barb nodded.

"That was me," she said.

Barb continued to want her smoking breaks and, with Pat not there when I visited that day, I was the biggest, strongest person around, so I had the job of moving her into her wheelchair. I didn't relish the task at first, afraid as I was that I might drop Barb or hurt her. Still, I dutifully jumped up to do it every time I was needed.

Barb's breath was foul. Often I caught a whiff from her urine bag and felt like retching. These odours repelled me, but that didn't seem important. Instead, I started to feel good that I was doing my bit.

I had always kept my professional distance, observing, probing, interviewing, judging. Now, I realized, I was doing a different kind of work. I couldn't live by the convenient and familiar rules. A greater responsibility was demanded. Of course, I was still required to ask the hard questions and to write down all that I saw and heard, but I had to do so without the benefit of distance. I had to do it up close. And, now, lifting up a dying friend into her wheelchair, pushing her to the smoking room, helping her wth her cigarettes, then wheeling her back and getting her settled in bed, I was there. I was doing it.

On her evening shift, Tracy read Barb the latest tabloids; Barb had always loved to hear the celebrity gossip. A few times, Barb woke up, smiled at her friend, and said, "I love you."

Just then, Tracy thought about how Barb was supposed to have died before Christmas. She turned to Barb, who was awake for a moment.

"Barb, it's May! Can you believe it?"

"I know," Barb nodded and grinned. "Hey!"

Sunday, May 4. The core group was starting to falter from exhaustion, as well as the disquiet of seeing Barb's deterioration, and the stress of not always knowing quite what to do to help her. Pat told me he'd gone without sleep for 42 hours straight. Dark shadows became a fixture around his eyes.

With Barb, he realized he was no doctor, so he didn't worry about her medical care, just her comfort. If she wanted to get up, he would get her up. Thirsty, get her a drink. Hungry, fetch her some food.

He tried to never despair about her condition. He told me he would end up in a rubber room if he went in that direction. With others, Barb always made an effort to be polite, but she could still be crabby with Pat. He said he didn't mind. In fact, he admired her for it. He'd always loved her fight.

Once, when he hauled up Barb to guide her into her wheelchair, she lay her head on his shoulder and smiled.

"We'll just stay here," she said.

Mackenzie came in every afternoon with Little Barb, but resisted being alone with her mom, retreating as quickly as she could to Unit 43's family room, where she would play the electric organ or do a puzzle.

"Just go in and tell her what you did that day, what you had to eat," Little Barb urged Mackenzie. "I know you don't like it sometimes, but it's important for you, and it's important to your mom. It means a lot."

But Mackenzie seemed uncomfortable around her mom. She feared something might happen if she was alone in the room with her. At the same time, when there were other people around, including Greg and me, she felt shy.

The nurses also had concerns about the great number of guests that came to see Barb, saying the constant bustle and visiting might be making it hard for her to settle. Greg was singled out as someone who was there more than almost anyone else.

Pat started to question his presence. Why did he always have to have his camera when he was visiting? Didn't he have enough pictures?

Tracy talked with me about the issue, and, in turn, I talked to Greg. He agreed it would be best to back off. In fact, he was relieved to get a break.

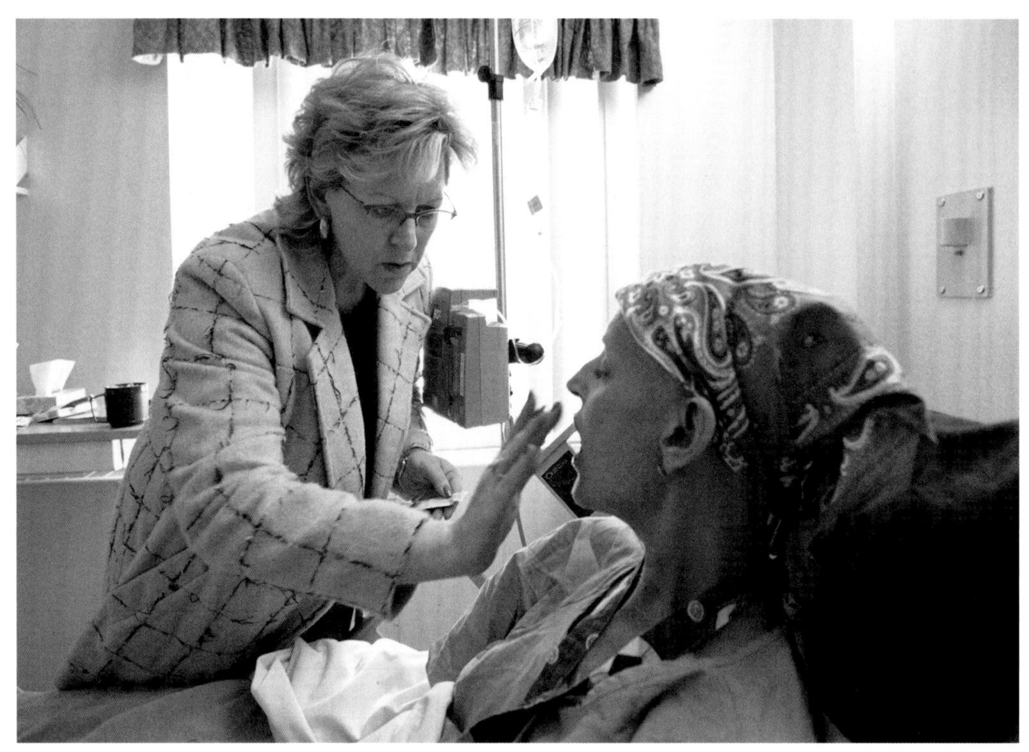

Tracy puts Vaseline on Barb's lips.

When I told Tracy the issue had been settled, she was much relieved, too. "I know there's a lot of stress going on," she e-mailed me, "and I don't want Pat or me or you or Greg or anyone to blow up one day over something that can be solved."

Monday, May 5. Barb now had her heart set on getting out on Wednesday for a visit home. In the morning, she got a hospital menu and circled every single food item, hoping to eat them all and gain strength.

Tuesday, May 6. A nurse was helping Barb to sit on the toilet, but turned away for a second. Just then, Barb crashed to the floor, landing on her knees, her head crashing into the door, bashing her nose, cutting her lip. Afterwards, she started to moan in her sleep from her pain.

Despite the injuries, she remained determined to get out of the hospital. A doctor cleared her to go out for a day trip, but told her it could happen only after a spell of unseasonably cold and snowy weather had ended.

When the doctor left the room, Barb tried to get up at once to leave.

"I can go," she told Pat.

"No, the doctor said later in the week when it warms up."

"Listen! Are you a fucking idiot! He said I can go."

"OK," Pat said. "I'm an idiot. But you can't go."

Barb turned to Little Barb. "You got to get me out of here."

"OK," Little Barb said. "I'll go down and get a lottery ticket and when you and I win on Thursday, I'll get a helicopter and get you out of here."

Barb started laughing.

In the end, Pat told her there was no way, between her injuries, the weather and her doctor's advice, that she was getting out, not at least until Friday.

Wednesday, May 7. In the smoking lounge, Barb flicked her lighter once, twice, three times, again and again, but could not get a flame going. When Tracy tried to help her by taking the lighter and holding it to Barb's cigarette, Barb got cranky, swatting away Tracy's hand.

This was typical of Barb's hard head, I thought. She had walked until she absolutely had to have a cane. She used the cane until she crashed down constantly and was forced into a wheelchair. She refused morphine until the agony was too great. She forced herself out of bed to go to schools, even when fatigue overwhelmed her. And now this, swatting away Tracy's hand. The indignant look on Barb's face made clear her thoughts: *I'm no invalid. I'll light my own cigarette, thank you very much.*

Thursday, May 8. In the morning, Tracy and her sister Jackie visited. Barb mumbled so much that Jackie couldn't understand a word she said.

Barb looked all crooked and scrunched in her bed. Tracy and Jackie straightened out Barb's body and got her a thick blanket. Barb fell asleep. A patch was put on her arm to help her with her nicotine cravings.

Greg and I visited in the evening, and got good news from Little Barb, who said Barb had been more settled that afternoon and had rebounded enough to visit with others again. She had sat up in bed, then called in Mackenzie, along with Mackenzie's cousins,

Little Barb's daughters, Ashley and Nicole. Barb held hands with the girls and had a long talk about what they had done that day and what they planned for the weekend. Barb gave Little Barb a list of what she would need for her own outing from the hospital, now planned for May 11, Mother's Day.

Mackenzie told her mom she was working on a Mother's Day present, a quilted wall-hanging with butterflies and dragonflies. She hoped it would make her mom feel at home.

At last, Mackenzie seemed relaxed around her mother.

Barb was asleep again when we arrived. We visited with Little Barb for about an hour and were about to leave when Barb awoke. Just as Little Barb had said, Barb seemed to be more focused and lucid.

Greg and I sat with her. At first, we made a bit of small talk, chatting about the coming episode of *Survivor*, a show that both Barb and I enjoyed. I told her that Frank Calder had said AADAC planned to run her ads for years to come because they had proven to be so effective.

I'd wanted to talk to Barb about what her crusade and her friendship had meant to me. I now had the chance, maybe my only chance. Still, I hesitated, fearful that my emotions would overwhelm me. At last, I breathed in and out heavily and started to talk. I told Barb that her work had done an incredible amount of good, and that I felt lucky to have been a part of it. "It was an honour to have been included," I said.

Barb mumbled in reply, and I couldn't understand all she said, but did make out one thing. "No," she said. "*I* am so lucky."

She tried to tell us that we'd helped her so much, and that we were responsible for much that she'd accomplished.

"Knock it off with the modesty," I said and laughed.

"You'd have done it all without us, Barbie," Greg said. "Of course, maybe it wouldn't have been quite the same."

She asked to hold our hands. I knew I had one more thing I needed to say. Barb had always called me and Greg her wee brothers. Now I felt like her real brother. I squeezed her hand.

"I love you, big sister," I said.

"Oh," she said, and mumbled something, I'm not sure what.

"I love you, too, Barb," Greg said.

We talked more about all the good she had done, and the fun times we had had, and what a great friend Tracy had been for her.

"You know what?" Barb said. "My time is here. And it's OK. It's OK."

I nodded. "Yes, I know Barb. It's OK."

She looked completely at peace.

We talked with her a bit more, about her injury, the bump on her head.

"I know!" she said. "I was mad, mad, mad, mad, mad, mad."

Just then, she started to look tired. Greg and I both said our good-bye for the night. She suddenly perked up. "You'll be back!?"

"Oh yes. We'll be here."

"Good," she said. "Good."

We left then. Both of us were elated and relieved. For months now, we had seen Barb meet others and put them at ease with her charm, her grace. Now she'd done it with us.

The gift of gab, I thought, a wonderful thing, yet not nearly so wonderful as the warmth of Barb, blarney and all.

Saturday, May 10. In the early morning hours, Barb had Tracy get her up out of bed, so she could go for a smoke. In the lounge, however, Barb was too tired to even lift her arms. Tracy lit a cigarette and held it to Barb's mouth. Barb tried to suck in the smoke, but couldn't do it.

Another smoker, a patient named Shelley Rhodes, who had come to befriend Barb, urged her on. "You can do it, Barb! You can do it."

Barb inhaled five quick times, but still couldn't draw in any smoke. She gave up.

It was her final cigarette.

Mother's Day, Sunday, May 11. The sun was bright and warm, and Pat was keen to take Barb on her outing. He got her out of bed and into the big reclining chair in her room, but that was as far as she wanted to go. Pat felt downcast. He knew how much she had wanted to get out, and what it meant that she couldn't. The cancer had sapped her.

"It used to be progressing at 40 miles an hour," he told Little Barb. "Since we got into the hospital, it's going 80 miles an hour."

Barb still tried to talk, but only a few words made any sense. Her breath started to rattle, so she was put on oxygen, a plastic vent placed under her nose.

"It's so hard to understand you these days," Little Barb told her that afternoon.

"A oke," Barb said. "A oke."

Little Barb shook her head. "We can't go for a smoke, the nurse said so. They just have you on oxygen, and you can't smoke."

Just then, Barb noticed the plastic vent under her nose and the tubes wrapped around her face. She moved to pull them off. Little Barb tried to stop her.

"Here, you stubborn person, keep it on."

But Barb insisted, still tugging at the tubes. Little Barb relented.

"Here, I'll get it off for you, but you're not going for a cigarette until Pat gets here to get you out of bed."

"Thanks," Barb mumbled, then drifted off to sleep, forgetting her urge to light up.

Monday, May 12. As a dying person weakens, the muscles in their face contract. Barb's jaw muscles pulled back on her chin. The skin around her eyes also drew tight, giving her face a cadaverous appearance. Her legs and arms were bone-thin. Her collarbone, spine and hip bones all protruded. Visitors who hadn't seen her in some time were shocked

She still tried to communicate, mumbling words. From the look in her eyes, it was clear she recognized and understood people. As much as anything, she appeared fed up with her disease, but was still fighting it, still ready to claw her way out of bed and give one more speech if she could. You could hear her mind working, sending out her message: *Look at me! This is what the cigarette does. Tell me, guys, how cool is this?*

Her eyes no longer sparkled, but still there was a spark. Barb had always said the cancer would never touch her spirit. It never did.

In the morning, Father Mike came in and gave Barb her last rites. He put his hands upon her head, praying in silence that the Holy Spirit would enter her and provide strength and perseverance. He anointed her forehead with holy oil, and said the Lord's Prayer. Barb said it with him, speaking more clearly than she had in days.

Shortly after Father Mike's visit, Dr. Pablo Amigo checked on Barb. In the hallway, he told Little Barb that Barb's heart and kidneys were still strong and functioning. "It's amazing considering how her condition is deteriorating so much. Now we're hoping for the best, preparing for the worst, and taking it one day at a time. We're making sure she's comfy. That's what we can do."

Barb slept almost all of the time, waking up only for a few moments now and then. During her shift, Tracy sat in the hallway outside of Barb's room, watching her as she slept. At times, she would go in and talk to Barb about what was coming next, and how she would soon see Patrick, Michael and Tracy's own brother Tim. She also read Barb a note that she'd written.

"I want you to know how much I love you," Tracy said. "I will miss you deeply, but know you will always be by my side. Thanks for being a special part of my life."

Tuesday, May 13. Barb needed some help with a denture plate, which had wedged itself into her mouth. Two nurses had tried and failed to get it out. Little Barb had also tried, and Barb almost bit off her finger.

Tracy now made an attempt. "I hope I don't hurt you," she said. "You want me to get them out, right?"

Barb moaned.

"Can you open your mouth?"

Barb opened it a bit. Tracy made a brief attempt, then noticed how shrivelled Barb's lips were.

"Want some water in your mouth, Barb? It looks pretty dry. I should get you some rye and coke."

Tracy took a sponge and dripped water into Barb's mouth. All the time Greg took pictures. I could see how powerful these images were going to be, as Barb's arms had pulled back reflexively and her hands had flopped inward, one more mark of approaching death.

Wednesday, May 14. I was keen to see Greg's pictures of Tracy and Barb from the previous day. He was uncertain about how they would turn out as the room had been quite dark. On his computer screen at the Journal office, Greg pulled up the images. A photograph of Tracy tending to Barb, Barb with her contracted arms and hands, came onscreen. We both gasped.

"Oh my God," I said.

At once, we looked away.

"Dave, I've got to shut this off," Greg said, turning off the computer. "It's too painful."

The overwhelming impact of the photograph was perplexing. We had both been in the room with Barb and Tracy when Greg took this picture. Everything had seemed normal. And yet, now, seeing an image of what I'd seen with my own eyes, I felt a great surge of emotion.

The image didn't look real to me. It wasn't the Barb I knew. She was so vulnerable. From the glazed look in her eyes, it seemed as if she was already gone.

Along with feelings of sadness, though, I felt revulsion, horror even, not at Barb's condition, but at the image itself.

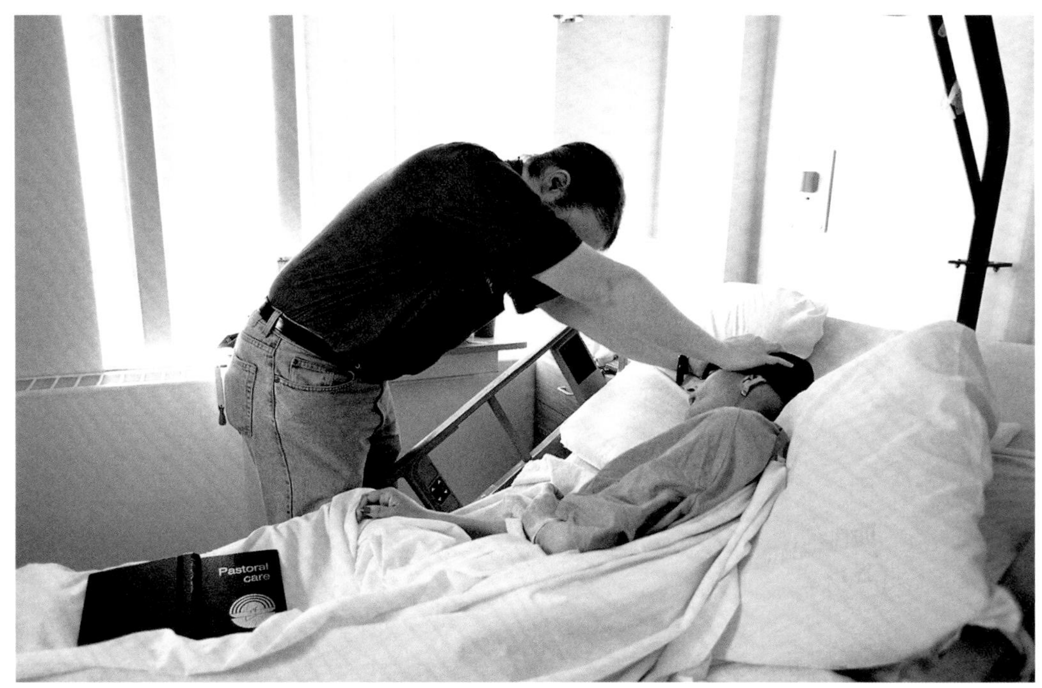

Barb receives the last rites from Father Mike Mireau on May 12.

This photograph should be destroyed, I thought. If it was too horrific for us to look at, surely no one else should see it either.

I mentioned this to Greg, but his instinct was that the photo had to run. Of course, he was right, I quickly realized. If the image had hit us that hard, it would have the same impact on others. It showed exactly how ugly and nasty things got for cigarette smokers. It was the picture that Barb had always wanted to be taken.

Greg's job was done now. He'd fulfilled his promise to Barb.

Thursday, May 15-Saturday, May 17. Little to report. Barb slept all day, not talking to anyone, not getting out of bed. She was down to 75 pounds.

Sunday, May 18. Barb's eyes remained tightly shut as she slept, but her breathing started to become more laboured, one long, loud breath, followed by two quick huffs, then silence for a long time, before the pattern repeated itself.

Cheyne-Stoking, the nurses called the raspy, irregular breathing pattern.

Rhymes with chain smoking, I thought.

When Susan Shaw came in for her night shift, she recognized that Barb was in her last stage and could die at any moment.

"Ah, shit, Barb!" Susan said just then. "I knew you were going to make me do this."

Like Tracy and Barb, Susan believed in dream prophecy, and she'd had a recurring dream where she took care of Barb in her final moments.

She got to work. She anointed Barb with holy water from Lourdes, dabbing it on her forehead in the sign of the cross. She said prayers, asking that Barb be with God in his eternal kingdom and that she would no longer have to bear the cross she'd carried any longer.

A Catholic herself, Susan recited the Rosary, making the sign of the cross, then starting out with the Apostles Creed: "I believe in God, the Father Almighty, Creator of heaven and earth; and in Jesus Christ, His only Son, our Lord. . ."

Susan also asked the nurses to go call Pat and Mackenzie, saying that they had better get down to the hospital very quickly. It was 11:00 p.m., and Pat had to make the drive from work at West Edmonton Mall.

A few moments later, Barb opened her eyes. She seemed to look into the distance, and it felt to Susan like she was trying to locate Michael in the mists of what was to come.

"Run to him," Susan said. "Go!"

Barb shut her eyes. A moment later, she was gone.

Saturday, May 24. I didn't bring a notebook to Barb's funeral. Greg left behind his camera, as well. We didn't want to go there as reporter and photographer, but as friends.

All week I'd been working on my final, major newspaper report on Barb, a 10,000-word story, describing her final months. I'd been thinking hard once again about what it had all meant. A huge weight still seemed upon me. In some ways, it had all been so despairing. At the same time, all of those closest to Barb felt at peace. We felt good that we'd all been able to properly say good-bye.

Still, I felt that weight was holding me back. It seemed as if something was missing in my under-

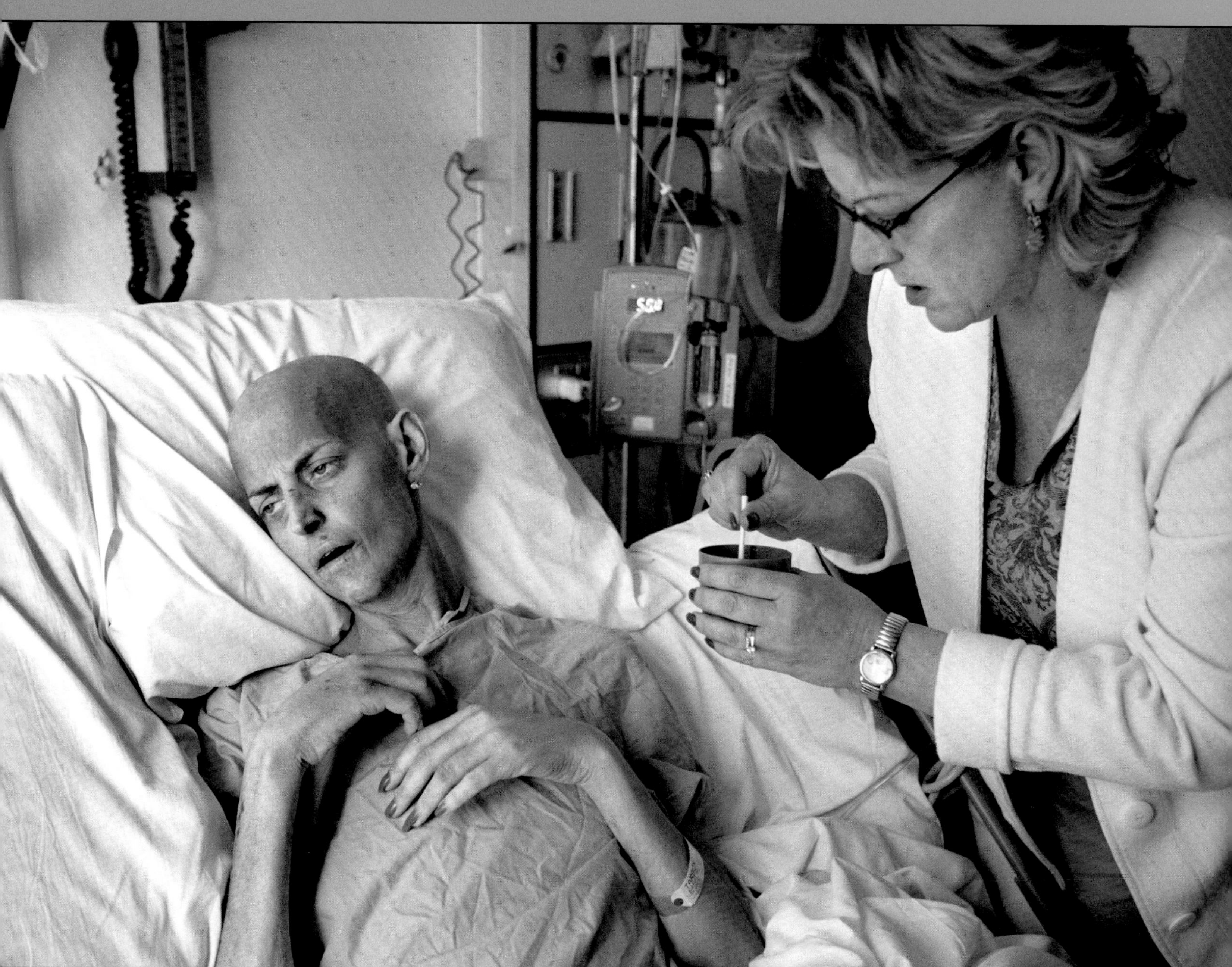

Tracy dabs Barb's lips with water. A moment later, Barb took a sip from the cup.

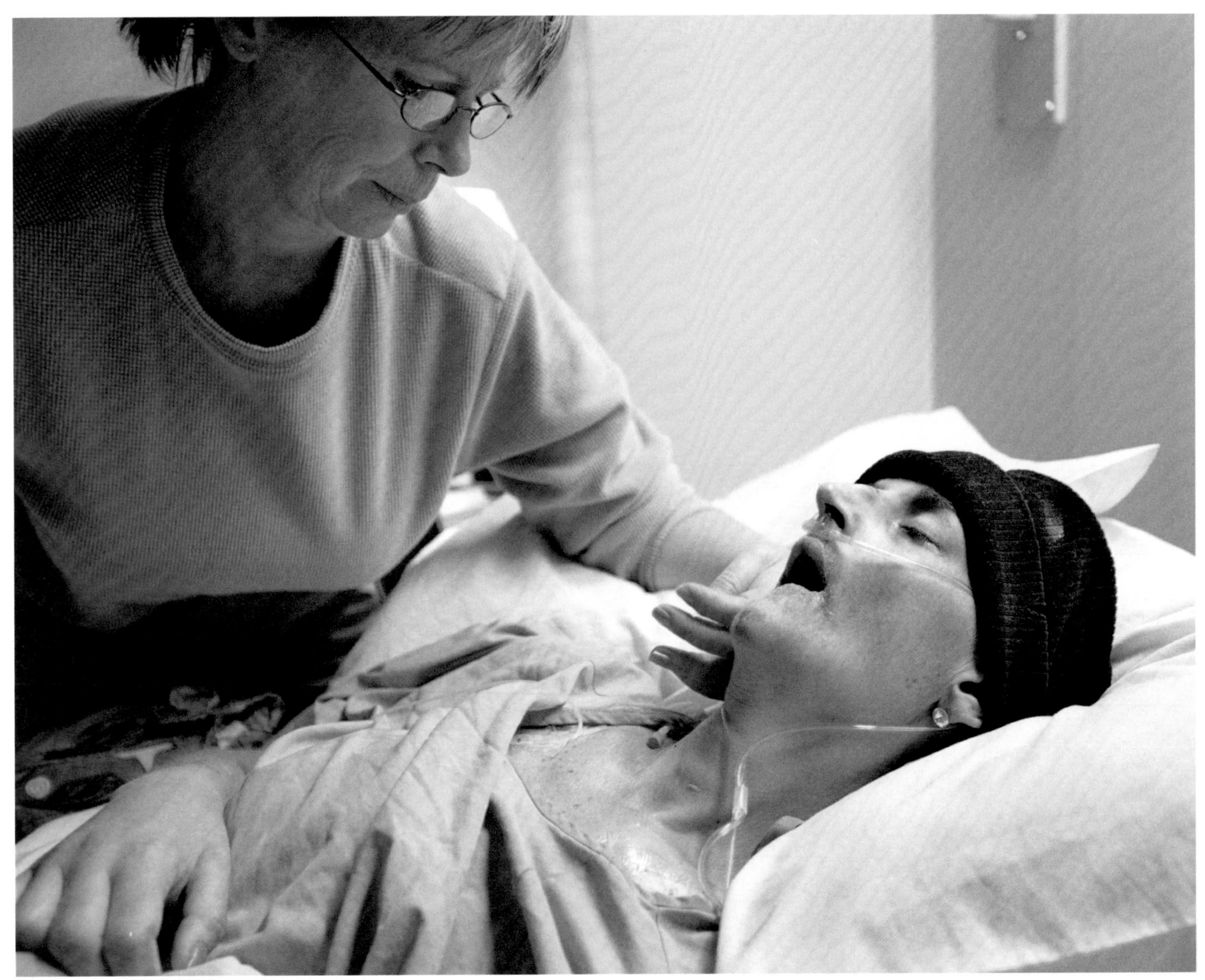

Susan Shaw comforts Barb by rubbing her face. This was May 14th, the last day Greg saw Barb.

standing of all that had transpired. I had yet to find the right words to describe what I had seen.

It was a warm, sunny day, late spring in Edmonton. Tracy bought dresses emblazoned with butterflies for both Miranda and Mackenzie. They played in front of the church as people filed in. Numerous dignitaries attended Barb's prayer service, then her funeral, including Federal Health Minister Anne McLellan, Provincial Health Minister Gary Mar, Lieutenant-Governor Lois Hole, Edmonton Mayor Bill Smith, and MP David Kilgour, who told reporters: "She's an icon. My father died of lung cancer after smoking for 30 years. There's no way on earth I wouldn't have been here to honour her."

I wasn't expecting much from the service. Most Christian funerals leave me unmoved, with their endless sermonizing about the need for repentance in order to ensure your place in heaven. But Father Mike Mireau, a young priest with glasses and a pony tail, gave a different kind of talk. He told the mourners about how he had first met Barb in November 2002, when she and Pat came in to plan her funeral and to get her confirmed in the Roman Catholic Church. Father Mike had been impressed with her spirit and generosity, how she wasn't one to hold back compliments. He could also see she liked to get her way.

Barb told Father Mike she was due to die in a few short weeks, at Christmas.

"Of course, Barb had something else in mind, and obviously God agreed," Father Mike said. "Now my job as a priest is to be able to recognize miracles. It's to recognize the different places that Jesus shows up in our lives. That's my job. Well, I think I've seen it. We've all come to know the story. We all know of the countless thousands whose lives have been touched by Barb Tarbox over the course of the last several months. What we have seen is Barb let God turn her into a miracle, and as priest I've come to firmly believe that what we've seen in Barb is an image of Jesus, that her mission, her suffering, and her love, became patterned on Jesus himself.

"Now Barb would be embarrassed to hear me say that. In fact, she probably is embarrassed. She wasn't perfect; she'd be the first person to admit that. . .What she was was someone who had made a mistake, a mistake that she deeply regretted, that she was furious at herself for, because that mistake would cost her her life, and take her away from her family. But she wasn't going to let it end there, and neither was God.

"Barb was going to die, she knew it. It was inevitable. What was so remarkable about her was the *way* in which she died. She turned her tragic and painful death into a way of speaking the truth about smoking. She allowed herself to become that truth, a living image of it, that smoking kills. . . She put her own suffering *on display*, so that people, especially children, would see it, that they would be shocked and saddened and broken-hearted by it, and they would stop smoking. And so many have. They have because Barb had the courage to take her suffering and *love people with it.* And so God gave her months and months and months to reach thousands and thousands and thousands with that love. And in Barb, we see God turning tragedy into triumph."

Father Mike concluded his address, restating his belief. "It's at this time of year, the Easter season, when we celebrate life coming from the death of our Lord, that we see the possibility of so many saved lives coming from Barb's own death. So I am willing to stand here and stake my reputation as a priest on my conviction that what we have witnessed in Barb is a miracle. It's God showing up in our lives, bringing triumph out of tragedy, bringing life out of death."

At that moment, listening to Father Mike, grieving Barb's loss, it seemed to me as if he were speaking factually, not fancifully. At last, someone had perceived the heart of Barb's crusade and was giving it its due. There was a rightness to Father Mike's ideas, poetic justice at least, if not a greater truth. He had found the concept that I had been searching for, the word to describe what transpired in the past months with Barb: *miracle.* I felt grateful.

May 18, 2004. I've now had almost a year to consider what Father Mike said about Barb's miracle. It's led to a more involved search about the nature of miracles themselves. The most enlightening book on the matter is Kenneth L. Woodward's excellent history, *The Book of Miracles: The Meaning of the Miracle Stories in Christianity, Judaism, Buddhism, Hinduism, Islam.*

Miracles aren't just the province of the Christian faith, Woodward writes, but are part of every important human faith. Moses divided the waters of the Red Sea to save his people. Jesus raised his friend Lazarus from the dead. The Prophet Mohammed blinded an opposing army with a handful of dust. Krishna lifted a mountain to save a village. The Buddha dazzled his kinfolk by rising in the air, dividing his body into pieces, then rejoining them.

Barb's miracle didn't involve anything so spectacular, unless, of course, you believe Father Mike's assertion that in her final days, Barb supernaturally took on the appearance of Christ and his mission. I can't claim to have seen this, but, upon reflection, I did see several things that hinted at the possibility that something unusual had come into play here.

If there is a God, I wouldn't expect the Maker's designs to be obvious and heavy-handed, but to be intricate and mysterious, baffling to most people until time and distance gave them the perspective necessary to comprehend. In my mind, two matters stand out from Barb's crusade that fit that definition.

The first is Barb's smoking. At first glance, I saw her ongoing smoking and preaching just as so many others did, as hypocritical. I later changed my own mind, but the issue forever dogged Barb. She got lambasted and she, herself, saw it as a failure and an embarrassment. In the end, though, something peculiar happened: Barb's smoking became the most powerful aspect of her anti-smoking crusade.

In June, shortly after Barb's death, when Pat, Mackenzie and I finally made that trip to New York to appear on the Montel Williams show, it was the story of Barb having her final smokes in palliative care that most moved Williams. More than that, the photographs that Greg took of Barb smoking in Unit 43 are the most haunting images of addiction that came out of the crusade. Long after what Barb said and did is forgotten, long after any other context of her work is stripped away, people will be able to look at these photographs and grasp their meaning at once: You smoke, you die.

The images should go on the side of every cigarette box in Canada: Here it is, the future, a few last drags before dying.

If Barb had done what most people thought was logical and reasonable for an anti-smoking crusader to do, if she'd quit her habit, her impact would have been far less powerful.

Instead, the greatest weakness of Barb's crusade became its greatest strength. It's a peculiar twist. It speaks of the possibility that her continued smoking was part of a greater design.

The second matter, the more important and convincing one, is Barb's motivation. As I've already said, I came to see her crusade as an act of atonement: Barb believed she had a debt to pay and she went about doing it by warning teenagers about smoking.

In time, this act rebounded; through her work, she discovered a way to beat back the self-loathing and loneliness that otherwise would have embittered her final months.

Maybe this plan of action came to her in a dream. Or maybe it derived from an intuitive sense of how to help herself. This is the explanation that I favour. The fact that Barb conjured up her own healing makes it no less astonishing to me than if a God had done it. If we accept a less lofty definition of miracle, and look at a miracle as merely a unique and mysterious act, something beyond normal explanation, then this was nothing short of one.

But perhaps there is another explanation for what happened, that Barb acted because she was on a God-directed mission, just as Father Mike and so many letter writers believed to be the case.

I don't know.

But, to me, it looked as if, during the desperate, madcap rush of her crusade, Barb stumbled upon her reward. At the start, she hadn't hoped for anything except to pay down her debt. As she got into her work, she realized that talking to the teens gave her energy, and momentarily took away her physical pain, but she never anticipated any greater relief than that. She never made the calculation that if she called herself the world's biggest idiot, and showed off her bald head, and wept, raged and hugged 50,000 school children, that she would have an overwhelming sense that she'd made good, and that God had forgiven her.

But with atonement came grace.

By hungering and thirsting to save others, Barb saved herself. By loving others, she found a way to forgive herself. It was a wonder to behold.

For Barb, it was a miracle.

Resources

International
World Health Organization (WHO)
Tobacco Free Initiative (TFI): http://www.who.int/tobacco/en/
Quit&Win2004: http://www.quitandwin.org

Canada
Health Canada
Tobacco Control Programme
http://www.hc-sc.gc.ca/hecs-sesc/tobacco/index.html or
http://www.gosmokefree.ca
Quitting:
http://www.hcsc.gc.ca/hecssesc/tobacco/quitting/index.html
Quit4Life (Q4L) (Youth/Quitting)
http://www.hc-sc.gc.ca/hecs-sesc/tobacco/youth/quit/quit.html
Canadian Lung Association
http://www.lung.ca
Quitting: http://www.lung.ca/smoking/smoking_cessation.pdf
Canadian Council for Tobacco Control (CTCC):
http://www.cctc.ca/
Physicians for a Smoke-Free Canada: http://www.smoke-free.ca/

Canadian Provinces
Alberta Alcohol and Drug Abuse Commission (AADAC)
http://www.barbtarbox.com
http://tobacco.aadac.com/
Calgary Health Region – Tobacco Reduction Youth
http://www.crha-health.ab.ca/pophlth/tobacco/youth.htm
British Columbia Ministry of Health Services
Tobacco Strategy:
http://www.healthplanning.gov.bc.ca/tobacco/index.htm
Tobacco Facts: http://www.tobaccofacts.org
Manitoba Department of Health
http://www.gov.mb.ca/health/index.html
Government of the Northwest Territories Health and Social Services
http://www.hlthss.gov.nt.ca/Features/Initiatives/initiatives.htm
Nova Scotia Department of Health Tobacco Control Unit
http://www.gov.ns.ca/health/tcu/default.htm
Government of Saskatchewan
http://www.health.gov.sk.ca/rr_smokeless_tobacco.html
http://www.health.gov.sk.ca/ps_tobacco_reduction.html
Saskatchewan Lung Association:
http://www.sk.lung.ca/smoking/
Yukon Department of Health and Social Services
http://www.hss.gov.yk.ca/prog/hp/tobacco/index.html

United States
Centers for Disease Control (CDC)
Health topic: Tobacco
http://www.cdc.gov/health/tobacco.htm
Tips for Youth
http://www.cdc.gov/tobacco/tips4youth.htm
Tobacco Information and Prevention Source (TIPS): I Quit
http://www.cdc.gov/tobacco/educational_materials/iquit.htm
National Cancer Institute (NCI)
Publication list https://cissecure.nci.nih.gov/ncipubs/
American Lung Association's Freedom from Smoking Program
http://www.lungusa.org/ffs/index.html
National Spit Tobacco Education Program: http://www.nstep.org

Quitting:
E-Quit — Online Cessation Program;
http://www.infotobacco.com
Quitnet — A Free Resource to Quit Smoking: http://www.quitnet.com/qn_main.html
Stop Smoking Center http://www.stopsmokingcenter.org
National Spit Tobacco Educational Program (NSTEP)
http://www.nstep.org/resources/cessation/users.html
QuitTobacco.com http://www.quittobacco.com/
What You Need to Know About Smoking Cessation
http://quitsmoking.about.com/
NoTobacco.org http://www.notobacco.org/

Youth and Smoking
A Breath of Fresh Air
http://www.4woman.gov/QuitSmoking/teens.cfm
National Center for Tobacco Free Kids http://www.tobaccofreekids.org/
Media Awareness Network http://www.media-awareness.ca/english/index.cfm
Health Canada: You and Me Smoke Free http://www.hc-sc.gc.ca/hecs-sesc/tobacco/youth/index.html

Pregnancy and Smoking
Pregnets Web site http://pregnets.org/

Editor's Note:

When we started the Books Collective in 1992, our goal was to publish new, special voices, voices of unusual people, of people who made a difference — and above all, of people who could bear witness to the truth in a special way.

When we heard about Greg and David's determination to bring Barb Tarbox's story into a book, we knew we wanted to be its publisher. Few 21st century Canadian voices so far have had as much impact as Barb Tarbox's ferocious cancer-motivated howl of warning against smoking. And Greg's photos and David's narrative were with her as she carried that crusade across the country and to tens of thousands of people — primarily youth, but in a message which cuts across generations.

We were delighted when Greg and David chose us over bigger publishers, household names in Canada, and we have done our best to honour Barb's intent as we worked with Greg, David, the designer, the printer and all the other people who make a book happen and get it out to its readers. We have worked with some remarkable partners in the process, but the most remarkable one is the one who isn't here.

Barb Tarbox died one year ago. Neither Timothy Anderson nor myself ever met her, except through Greg's photos and David's newspaper stories, and then this book. Yet in the end, she exacted her share of tears from us too. We accepted from the beginning that no meeting, no planning or editing session, was complete without the box of Kleenex. It wasn't possible to keep our distance — nor should it ever be.

Tears are mentioned a lot in this book, enough that they almost sound like a badge of accomplishment. They are, but the accomplishment in this case is Barb Tarbox's. She was dedicated, honest, and loving enough to send the truth like a spear to our protected modern hearts — and when we are struck by truth, tears are the mark of our surrender.

Our defenses are breached, and when that happens, we cry. Not the crocodile tears of podium celebrities but the real, nasty, sinus-stinging tears of recognition and grief. Some see tears as a sign of weakness. But really, they are a sign of strength — the strength to listen to the truth, and accept that we have something more to learn: about ourselves, each other, our humanity; about how courage and kindness in the midst of our human imperfection are not saintly, not abstract, but personal and possible.

Barb's truth was an ugly one: she was dying of an ugly disease caused directly by an ugly personal and social addiction to a drug more powerful than heroin. She wanted youth to know: she made Greg and David promise not to flinch; she supported them in their coverage and insisted they complete this book. True to their promise, Greg and David have been dedicated, honest, and perhaps even brutal enough to keep rubbing that truth in our faces, keeping a promise to Barb to make her death as ugly as it really was. Yet like the miracle David describes Barb undergoing, there's a miracle they have performed as well. They have shown us beauty in the midst of that ugliness, great love in the midst of pain.

Barb spoke directly to kids. At one point Pat advised her, and she decided, as David recounts, that she was not going to get involved in the politics of smoking. This book doesn't talk about the way cigarettes are spiked with toxic substances to increase their addictiveness, and peddled by global corporations to children for profit. It talks instead about a brave, loving woman in that addiction's grip who couldn't get out of its coils but who could make her life — and her death — count for others. This book doesn't suggest remedies or panaceas, be they legal, medical or institutional. It's not that those wouldn't be worthy, but this is not a book about prescriptive answers.

It is a book about the life work of Barb Tarbox, a remarkable — and truly human — person who made her humanity, her limitations, her weaknesses, into her strength — and then gave it to others so that we could benefit from the loss she and those she loved suffered. That is an act of love both great and humbling.

So in a way, and in every way, this is a book about love. From Barb's heart through our work into your hands and thoughts. We hope you pass it on.

Candas Jane Dorsey
for River Books
an imprint of The Books Collective

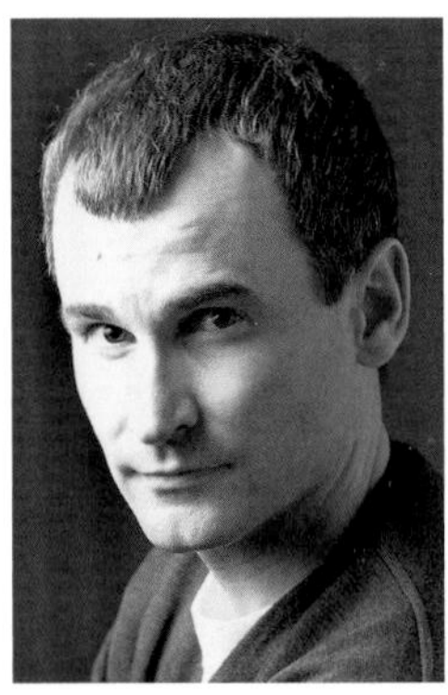

Greg Southam has worked at the Edmonton Journal since 1988. Southam has received numerous awards for his photojournalism over the past 20 years.

In 2001, he was awarded two National Newspaper Award certificates of merit for sports photography, making him the first photographer to receive two awards of such distinction in the same category in one year.

Further to that, Greg was named Canadian Sports Photographer of the Year, and thus joined an elite league of photographers and journalists in Canada who have been recognized for their outstanding work in the news industry.

Southam has also been nominated for a National Newspaper Award for feature photography and a photojournalism award presented by the Canadian Association of Journalists, both for his documentary work on Barb's story.

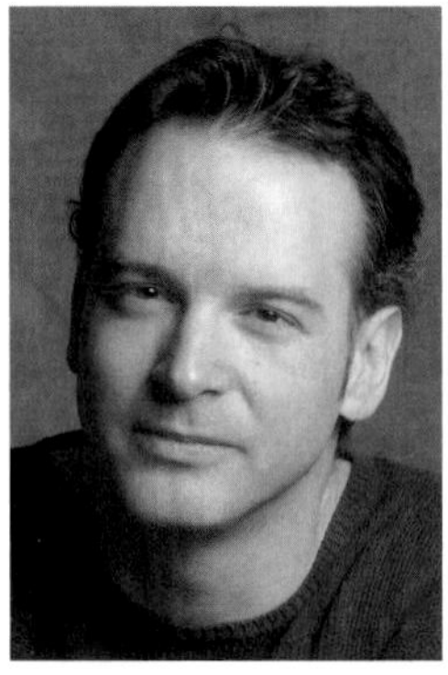

Writer David Staples is the best-selling co-author of the 1995 non-fiction thriller, *The Third Suspect: Inside the Hunt for the Yellowknife Mine Murderer*, the story of the 1992 Northwest Territories gold mine strike, mass murder and RCMP investigation. "Crime writing at its best," author Martin O'Malley said of the book. "Deserves a Pulitzer."

In 2002, Staples' profile on Worldcom CEO and accused fraud artist Bernie Ebbers of Mississippi was selected by *New Yorker* editor James Surowiecki for the Best Crime Writing of the Year book.

A veteran columnist at the Edmonton Journal, Staples has won a National Newspaper Award and two National Magazine awards.

He is married to writer and editor Lily Luong Ha Nguyen Staples and has four children, Jack, Ned, Joe and Daniel.